INTERMITTENT FASTING:

A COMPREHENSIVE GUIDE ON HOW TO LOSE WEIGHT AND KEEP IT OFF WITHOUT DIETING

I0449691

VIKTORIA WALDORF

TABLE OF CONTENTS

Introduction

This guide is to help you decide which fasting protocol is best for you and to help you understand how it works, the common myths, struggles and benefits, as well as guidelines for practices that can aid you in fasting and help you to be successful if and when you choose to endeavor into the program of intermittent fasting.

It will discuss different types of fasting and why Intermittent fasting is a good choice for you.

The information provided here is centered on how Intermittent fasting works. Of course, when you are considering changing the way you nourish your body and want to make a big change in your life, it is important to do so intelligently.

Intermittent fasting is not a new concept but it has recently become more widely used, and I wanted to put this book together to help you along this newly chosen path.

Chapter 1: What is intermittent fasting

Intermittent fasting simply means not eating for a designated period of time or a set number of hours and then eating during a time restricted feeding period. While the act of fasting has been around thousands of years, in the last several years, more and more women are engaging in the lifestyle of intermittent fasting. Intermittent fasting is proving to be highly beneficial to women health. There are countless benefits to participating in the lifestyle. Unlike the traditional diet, it focuses more on when you eat as opposed to what you eat. There are many ways to use fasting to your benefit and various techniques.

There is evidence of benefits on many body systems including slowing down aging, better cardiac health, better focus, weight loss, and multiple other benefits. While the vast majority of women are interested in intermittent fasting for the aid in weight loss, this guide goes over the other perks of the lifestyle, as well. Unfortunately, there is some negative stigma surrounding intermittent fasting.

Intermittent fasting can best be described as utilizing alternating intervals of fasting and feeding. The idea behind it is that you eat whatever you want, whenever you want during the feeding stage and avoid in taking anything with caloric value when in the fasting stage. We will discuss exactly how this affects your body and what the best practices are.

Intermittent fasting is a pattern of eating where you allocate specific hours in a day for eating and spend the rest of the day abstaining from food.

Here is a simple example of intermittent fasting. You eat your dinner by 7 pm in the evening and then go to bed. When you wake up, you don't eat any breakfast. You wait until around 10 am before you eat anything. The period between 7 pm and 10 am is your fasting window.

You are then allowed to eat anything you want between 10 am and 7 pm that evening. This is known as your "feasting" window. If you choose to exercise, you can do so before you begin your feasting period. It is important to note that during your fasting period, you can drink water and consume non-caloric beverages. Anything that contains sugar or alcohol should definitely be avoided.

As you can see, there are no major complications like having to drastically change your diet or eat lettuce all day. All you are required to do is stick to the feasting window you have chosen. You are the one who gets to choose the timings of your feasting and fasting windows. This adds to the flexibility of this technique.

Intermittent fasting involves alternating cycles of eating and fasting. There are quite a few studies that show that this can result in weight loss, protect against disease, improve metabolic health, and perhaps even help you live a longer life. As a woman, however, fasting can lead to hormonal imbalances or even fertility issues so we must ensure that we utilize intermittent fasting properly.

There are several different methods of intermittent fasting that you may choose from, and most people tend to start with lower alternating periods and slowly increase them. Intermittent fasting is actually fairly easy, and many people report having more energy and feeling better overall during their fasting periods.

Of course, many of us ignore our body's signals in an attempt to lose weight only to end up binge eating and then follow that with under eating, starvation, and binging again. A cycle like this can wreak havoc with your hormones, halt ovulation, affect your menstruation, and even shrink your ovaries. On top of that, it can exacerbate eating disorders, such as; bulimia, anorexia, and binge eating.

However, that does not mean you cannot enjoy the benefits of fasting. There are several different methods for intermittent fasting that we will review and discuss in a later chapter, including an alternative choice that helps your body more easily adapt to fasting and enjoy the benefits without accidentally causing your hormones to go crazy.

Chapter 2: The History of Intermittent Fasting

Fasting has been around nearly as long as mankind itself. There are many old written sources that have shown that "starvation" has been used in various cultures, countries, and ancient civilizations to help the body recover and restore itself. It seems they were taking advantage of the benefits long before modern times. Ancient India, Greece, and Rome, in particular, used intermittent fasting, not only to strengthen the body but also to help prevent diseases. Back in ancient times, when hunting and berry gathering was one of the main sources of food, there were periods of time where nothing could be found, so natural fasting took place. Involuntary fasting caused the hunters and gatherers to be inadvertently and greatly strengthened by the gaps in sustenance. The ancient Greeks particularly believed medical treatments and cures could be found and were observed in nature. When humans, dogs, cats, and most animals are sick, they do not want to eat. This is considered the internal physician in some cultures; it is believed that the body is instinctually fasting to help to heal its self. The ancient Greeks also believed fasting helped to improve mental and cognitive function. This makes sense if you think about when you eat a big meal and feel sleepy and tired or have "food coma" as many like to call it, versus when you are fasting and your brain hyper-focuses on the task at hand. The practices of controlled starvation are key in many of the world's religions, proving self-control, and penitence. Many religions practice fasting for periods such as Ramadan in the Islamic culture where they do not eat from sunup to sundown. Christianity recognizes the forty days of lent, which represents the time that Jesus Christ fasted. Fasting is recognized in Islamic religions, Buddhism, Christianity, and countless others.

Ramadan is an Islamic tradition that is practiced by Muslims. During Ramadan, they fast during the daylight hours, finally eating only once the sun has set. While it sounds terrible at first, many reports they actually feel better after a few days of the practice. This is because they adjust to the schedule and their bodies learn to adapt to no food for a time period. This is exactly what intermittent fasting is about.

However, in more recent years, there has been scientific research discovering and confirming the various benefits of intermittent fasting for women. Science is now beginning to prove what was already known in ancient times. The multiple and seemingly endless benefits keep climbing. The benefits include slowing down the aging process, sharper focus, weight loss, better cardiac health, there is evidence it both reduces the chances of cancer and helps your body to fight it off and a wide range of other advantages, with little consequences to the practice.

Chapter 3: Get Started with the Intermittent Fasting

You've got everything you need now to get started losing weight, feeling better, and getting healthier using intermittent fasting. All you have to do now is start!

Evaluate your current health and your goals.

Start by looking at your overall health as it currently stands. If you have any special concerns (like diabetes or other medical and health issues), review your new intermittent fasting intentions with your doctor to be sure you're healthy enough to begin. Determine how much weight you want to lose and set a realistic completion date. Once you begin practicing intermittent fasting and monitoring the speed at which you drop pounds, you can alter your goal and your completion date or incorporate an exercise routine to speed up your weight loss.

Identify which method of intermittent fasting will work best for your lifestyle and goals.

Read through the important information about each method of intermittent fasting. Consider your schedule, your lifestyle, and what you think might be easiest for you. You may consider trying a few different methods before deciding on the one that will be most effective for you. Remember, with each method, you can customize the fasting and eating hours to fit your preferences and schedule. The time of day of your fasting and when you eat is not what's important, so plan to break your fasts on days and during hours that will be convenient and easiest for you to stick to.

Start!

Once you've decided on a method you're ready to start. Keep a journal or a log of the times and days you plan to fast and when you'll be eating. This can help to keep you on track when you start, but won't be necessary for the long term. Your body will adjust to your new pattern of eating, and your hunger signals will soon be all the reminder you need that it's time to break your most recent fasting cycle!

Monitor your weight loss and incorporate an exercise routine for faster results.

If you're perfectly happy with the amount of weight intermittent fasting provides you per week, you may decide not to add a daily exercise routine. One of the goals of intermittent fasting is to reprogram these hormones and regulators back to their original state. This way, your body will send hunger signals when it's truly in need of nutrition—something, many women can't even remember experiencing!

It's as simple as that. As promised, intermittent fasting really is the weight loss strategy that can be adapted to anyone's lifestyle or goals. No special diet is required, and no lengthy exercise program is needed, but both can certainly be incorporated to boost your total weight loss.

Chapter 4: How to Stay Motivated When Using Intermittent Fasting

The first couple of weeks of intermittent fasting can not only be hard as heck, but it can also sometimes be a little disappointing if you don't see any physical results from your hard work. This can make it almost impossible for some women to stay motivated, especially if they actually see the scale go *up* in those first uncomfortable weeks.

Find a fasting buddy

It is easier to keep going when you know there is someone else fasting with you. It can be your husband, best friend, or family member. Sit down with them and walk them through the basics of the intermittent fasting technique you have chosen. Use each other as support on those days when one of you doesn't feel like fasting or exercising. It will be more fun when you have someone who you can plan meals with, shop for food with, train with and learn with. If you have someone else who is invested in your success, you won't want to do anything to let them down.

Set achievable goals

It is best to start with short-term goals that you know you can achieve. Once you attain that goal, reward yourself, but don't do it with junk food. Get a massage or buy some new workout clothes. This will help boost your momentum and motivation.

Keep a progress journal

This is a great way to look at the positive changes you have been experiencing ever since you started your fast. Get a diary and start writing how you feel and all the progress you are making. It is important to take time to look at how your body and life is transforming. Look at how your clothes fit, the energy you now have to play with your kids, and the way your sleep has improved. Track your positive progress and whip out that journal whenever you feel yourself losing motivation.

Don't beat yourself up

Yes, there are days when you will fail and succumb to temptation. Things will get rough, and you will grab a cookie and start munching away. Be compassionate with yourself. Don't start talking negatively about yourself just because you didn't do things right. The important thing is to get back up and keep going.

Pray and meditate

When you start to feel discouraged, take some time to feed and strengthen your soul and spirit. Pray, read scriptures, and meditate. This will help you love yourself despite the challenges you face in life.

Focus On the Good

Throughout the first few weeks I'm betting that you've found yourself with more energy, especially following the feeding phase, had heightened alertness, euphoria, and even creativity. That felt *great* didn't it? You've likely also had more time on your hands recently, particularly so if you are skipping a meal that you normally would spend a bit of time preparing. What does that extra time allow you to do? While you may not notice significant observable weight loss within those first days and weeks of intermittent fasting, there is always good point you can focus on. Think about the extra time that you're getting with your family or loved ones, all the extra stuff you're getting done, and how it's helping you at work to stay motivated when you're not seeing those quick results that you were hoping for. Usually, after week three or four is when you start to see the beginning of fat loss, and it's generally pretty steady from there.

Go slow

The success of a diet depends on the lifestyle changes that you decide to make. These changes take a while and they do not happen overnight. If you want to lose weight and make sure that it stays at bay, then you'll need to lose weight slowly. You can starve yourself and shed a few pounds, but it will not do you any good. The more gradual and steady your weight loss, the easier it is to maintain. Intermittent fasting is a great dieting option and it is sustainable. Make sure you go slowly. There is no hurry, and you don't need to jump right in.

Be Your Personal Coach

You are the best person to motivate yourself. You can program your mind to think precisely what you want it to think. You need to drive yourself by positively reinforcing your efforts and reminding yourself of your motivational reasons. Look at yourself in the mirror and say to your reflection (out loud) that you can overcome your food cravings and that you are doing this for your health. Each day, you can program your mind and body to become an incredible fat burning machine. When you use these self-motivational methods, your brain will believe everything you tell yourself. If you think you are going to fail, you will inevitably fail. But, if you genuinely think that you will succeed, you will succeed!

Be Willing to Forgive Yourself

Don't forget, Intermittent Fasting is not a walk in the park. You may realize it's not as easy as people make it out to be. There are going to be times when you slip up and make a mistake. Perhaps you choose to attend a birthday party, and in the process, you ate delicious food instead of sticking to your fasting schedule. That's absolutely fine. Just remember, do not beat yourself up about it because this is normal and you're only human. Instead of punishing yourself, realize the mistake, and immediately get back on track and move forward.

Setbacks are common

Temptation can strike and there will be times when you might give in to your temptations. There is no harm in this, and once in a while, it is okay. After all, you are only human. It is okay to face a setback, but don't think of it as a failure. The attitude with which you deal with a setback can set the course for the rest of your diet.

Don't try to be a perfectionist

So, what would you do if you polished off a bag of Oreos? Perfectionist thinking gets in the way of success more than any other factor. If a 200-calorie indulgence is just that, "an indulgence" and nothing more, then it's okay. However, if you perceive it as a failure and a reason to give up, it can quickly turn into a 1000-calorie indulgence. Don't try to be a perfectionist when you start to diet. As mentioned in the previous tip, setbacks are expected and you should deal with them in a positive way.

Be patient

One of the significant obstacles to a diet is the weight loss plateau. You might eat right and exercise correctly, but the numbers on the scales don't seem to change. The scale appears to be stuck for some reason. Well, this is known as the weight-loss plateau, and it is something that every dieter faces. Merely turn around and congratulate yourself for your success so far. It is a part of the process of weight loss.

Reward yourself

Dieting does take some effort, and it might not seem fun at times. So don't forget to treat yourself when you achieve a goal. A goal could be big or a small. It could be something as simple as avoiding sugary treats for a day. When you achieve your goal, you should treat yourself. The reward doesn't have to be an extravagant one. Perhaps you can buy yourself a bottle of nail polish that you wanted! The rewards you set for yourself should never be food related. Don't reward yourself with a pint of ice cream for losing 5 pounds in ten days. It doesn't make any sense and renders the diet redundant. When you celebrate your success, it will make you feel better about yourself and your diet. Also, it will provide you with the necessary motivation to keep going even when you want to give up.

Chapter 5: Benefits of Intermittent Fasting

Intermittent Fasting when there is an oscillation between periods of eating and fasting. There are several benefits offered by this diet and there are scientific studies as well as research that support these claims. In this section, we will cover the different benefits this diet offers.

Change in Cell Function

When you fast for a while, different changes take place in your body. For instance, your body will start a process of cellular repair and there will be changes in your hormone level. A difference in these levels makes it easier for the body to access the stored fat. You will notice that there is a reduction in the level of insulin and it helps increase the body's ability to burn fat. An increase in the human growth hormone helps to increase lean muscle and burn more fat than usual.

Weight Loss

The most obvious benefit of this diet is weight loss. When you follow intermittent fasting, the number of meals you eat will be reduced. When you eat less, the calories you consume will decrease as well. When the levels of insulin decline, growth hormone increases along with an increase in norepinephrine, which helps the body break down stored fat to provide energy. There is an increase in your metabolic rate when you fast, which helps the body burn more calories. The effect of intermittent fasting is two-fold. On the one hand, it increases your metabolic rate and therefore makes your body more efficient while burning fats. The reduction in the level of food you consume reduces your overall calorie intake. Both these conditions promote weight and fat loss. Also, most of the fats that your body burns come from the abdominal area. The fat in the abdominal region happens to be the most stubborn of all, which is why this diet is perfect for belly flab.

Make Your Skin Glow

Many people that have introduced Intermittent Fasting into their lifestyles have reported positive effects on their skin.

Reduce Stress

Free radicals are produced by our bodies when we breathe. A decent and healthy level is fine, as they stimulate repair. However, when our body produces more than it should, it can damage our cells which is called oxidative stress. It is one of the factors for aging skin, wrinkles, and graying hair.

Reduce Inflammation

One of the main reasons for inflammation is excessive free radicals in your body resulting in cellular damage. When our cells' mitochondria's (the powerhouse in our cells that give us energy) are damaged, they begin to release excessive free radicals. These, in turn, result in inflammation and DNA damage. All these problems vanish when you allow your body to be in a fasted state for extended hours.

Improve Your Brain's Health

Intermittent Fasting improves processes that are very crucial for our brain health. It can lead to reduced inflammation, reduced oxidative stress, reduced blood sugar levels and increased insulin resistance. It also helps to increase the levels of a brain-driven neurotropic factor, a brain hormone whose deficiency is linked to depression and other similar problems of the brain.

Increased Metabolic Rate

Without getting into the biochemistry of metabolism, it will be suffice to say that when you stretch out your eating schedule, as when you do when you practice intermediate fasting, your body increases its metabolic rate. The body is designed to operate effectively and efficiently when it runs on a lean diet. When it eats too much, the body needs to spend a lot of its time digesting food and shuttling it to various areas and, when in excess, has to convert it to fat and store it.

Mental Acuity and Strength

To keep you in a state of rest, the shot of hormones places your mind in a relaxed state and that reduces your mental acuity. It's primal in its design. Cavemen that needed to go out and hunt were given the extra boost in mental acuity and strength when they were hungry but turned sleepy and relaxed after a full meal. We, today, are no different. It has been researched and observed that intermittent fasting accelerates and prolongs the neural development in the brain.

Intermittent fasting stimulates the release of Brain-Derived Neurotropic factor (BDNF). This is a hormone instrumental in motivating the body and staving off any form of depression. When expressed periodically, it can boost your abilities. When expressed continuously, it will change your life.

Reduced Oxidation and Aging Stress

It is now well documented that the oxidation leads to things like heart disease and stroke by leading to the hardening of arteries and blood vessels. Oxidative stress also alters gene expression and the regulation of tissue repair. That has a direct impact on how your cells age as you want them to be flexible and elastic. That results in better looking skin and, when you do lose weight your skin will not sag because it is properly nourished.

Reduced Risk of Heart Disease

Intermittent fasting improves LDL levels, which has a direct impact on cardiovascular health. That, in turn, has an impact on blood pressure which is directly responsible for kidney health. This is done in two ways. First of all, it reduces the stress in your heart to keep working at digesting large quantities of food and storing energy in the fat cells. If you use what you take in, there is no need to put your heart through that stress. Ask anyone who is out of shape and on the larger side of life, how they feel after a meal – they will tell you they need to rest. Many need a cup of coffee. The coffee is to get caffeine into your system and push blood to your brain so that you get the energy you need. A better way would be to not eat so much. Don't look to be full and don't look to be satiated.

Repair Your Cells

Fasting can lead to autophagy, which is a cellular process for removal of waste. This entails cells breaking down and metabolizing dysfunctional, broken proteins, which build up in cells over extended periods of time. During this autophagy, your body builds protection against several diseases like Alzheimer's disease and cancer.

Lower the Risk of Diabetes

The most common health problem that plagues humanity these days, apart from obesity, is diabetes. High blood sugar leads to insulin resistance in the body. Intermittent fasting helps to reduce blood sugar and therefore helps reduce insulin resistance in the body. When your body becomes resistant to insulin, it leads to an increase in the blood sugar level and the vicious cycle goes on and on. If you opt for this diet, you can successfully reverse this condition.

Chapter 6: Things to Expect

It is easy, once you get into the groove

It is easy to follow the diet once you get into your fasting groove. You can start your day with a cup of unsweetened tea or coffee. Then keep yourself busy with work until noon. At noon, you can have your first meal and make sure that you eat health. Your body is used to a specific diet or rather no diet up until now, and therefore it will take a while for you to get used to intermittent fasting. Fasting isn't that difficult, and it does get easier with time.

Hunger Pangs

There is a lot of debate about breakfast being the most important meal of the day. The method of fasting that you opt for is entirely up to you. Hunger pangs are quite common during the initial week of fasting; don't get scared. Your body isn't used to fasting, and it will take a while to condition yourself to the diet. A hunger pang doesn't always indicate hunger. Confusing isn't it? At times, you will feel hungry when you are stressed or even bored. It is essential that you realize the difference between actual hunger and a natural craving. Ignore these pangs and get on with your day. Intermittent fasting doesn't mean that you should starve yourself, but at the same time, you shouldn't indulge in mindless eating either.

Benefits of exercise

When you exercise on an empty stomach you can burn more fat than you usually do. If weight loss is your primary goal, then you should try to exercise on an empty stomach. However, make sure that you don't take up any extreme forms of exercise. Even yoga on an empty stomach will increase your gains. When you exercise on an empty stomach, your body makes use of the stored fat to provide energy, and therefore it burns additional fat.

Change of perspective

Your perspective on food will change when you follow this diet. When you pay attention to what you eat and when you eat it, you will eat a whole lot healthier than ever before. The diet will make you conscious of the things you feed your system. When you eat healthier, you will feel better, and your energy levels will increase.

The scale might not take a nosedive

During the initial couple of days of the fast, the scale might not make a nosedive. The weight you lose depends on several factors like your diet, metabolism, and age. You will lose some weight, but don't be disheartened if it isn't at the rate that you thought it would be. The weight loss is gradual, and you'll need to be patient. Patience and consistency are critical when it comes to Intermittent fasting. Don't give up on the diet just because you didn't drop thirty pounds in thirty days. Instead, give it some time, stick to the diet, and see for yourself. You cannot lose weight overnight. If you think you can, then you are merely setting yourself up for failure.

Now that you know what to expect on your new diet, you will be better prepared to manage it with success.

Chapter 7: When and What to Eat

In this section, you will learn about when and what to eat when you fast. If you know the answer to this, then you can make the most of intermittent fasting. There aren't any hard and fast rules about intermittent fasting, and one of the best features of this diet is the flexibility that it offers. You can eat the food that you like, and you won't feel that you are on a constant "diet." The phrase "food you like" doesn't refer to all sorts of unhealthy treats and you should show some prudence when it comes to what you eat.

When to eat on a fast day?

For a lot of people, fasting all day long and having a good meal in the evening is the best plan for a fast day. If your calorie allowance is around 500 calories on a fasting day, then you can have one meal that's worth 500 calories at the end of the day. You also have the option of having mini-meals all through the day as long as you stick to the calorie restriction. If you follow the crescendo method of fasting, then you will fast on two or three days of the week and eat like you usually would on all the other days. On the days that you fast, you can eat after your fasting window ends. It means that you can eat after you complete 12-16 hours of fasting. After you break your fast, you can have a light meal and follow it later with one or two meals. As mentioned, there are different forms of fasting that you can follow so select one that suits your needs. If you like to have a heavy dinner, then you can save up your calories from the rest of the day and indulge yourself at night. A lot of people find it easier to wait until the evening to have a proper meal. If you fall into this category, then do so.

When you fast, you can have a couple of calorie-free snacks or maybe one low calorie bite, if you want. If you think you can do without the snack, then please do so! When you fast throughout the day, you might notice that your body is running low on fuel. In such a case, you can have a salty snack like a handful of popcorn! You can have a small bite during your fast, and it will not break your fast if you are careful about what you choose. Make sure that you drink plenty of water throughout the day. You can include a couple of cups of herbal tea or broth as well.

You'll need to remember that with intermittent fasting you can make your own rules. If you think you cannot fast all day long, you don't have to. You might like to have dinner and breakfast the following day, then you can. You don't have to worry about breaking any rules here. It is up to you and your comfort level.

What to eat on a fast day?

How can you make the most of your meals on a fast day? If all you can eat on a fast day is 500 calories, then make sure that you have as much protein and fiber as you can. If you follow a method of crescendo fasting or Lean gains method, then make sure that you eat at least 1200 calories and don't go beyond 15oo calories. You can have two hearty meals within this calorie restraint. You shouldn't be afraid to fill yourself up with lean proteins like fish, eggs and chicken. You can even have lots of salad and vegetables. It is quite easy to fast once you get used to it.

Popcorn - 25g of air-popped popcorn cooked in 5ml of coconut oil will garner you around 140 calories. The crunch of popcorn can also help alleviate cravings and help get you through snack time without banging your head against the wall trying to decide what to eat.

Nutella & Banana Rice Cakes - For a quick and easy snack that's around 200 cal just put a thin smear of Nutella on 2 rice cakes and top with a thinly sliced banana and you can even have an ice-cold cup of skim milk with this snack.

Kiwi & Red Capsicum - Slice a single kiwi and a red bell pepper for a simple snack that's less than 100 cal.

Mashed Cauliflower - Simply steam some cauliflower and mash it all up for a low-cal, low-carb, and tastier alternative to mashed potatoes.

Lettuce Leaf Wrap - Barely 100 cal and oh-so-easy to make. Just take 50g of chicken breast, 25g of grated zucchini, 25g of grated raw carrot, and wrap it all up in 1 leaf of Cos/Romaine lettuce.

Coconut Oil - Ten grams of refined coconut oil only have around 90 calories, and since it is processed by the liver as opposed to being stored as fat like many other oils, it's almost an instant energy boost. Since it is odorless and tasteless, you can add coconut oil to just about anything low-cal to give yourself a little extra pep in your step. Try adding some to your favorite low-cal yogurt, on a salad, mixed with scrambled eggs, or even smeared on a cracker. You'll be surprised at the difference this little trick can make.

How to manage a healthy fasting?

When it comes to foods, the best things to have around are:

- All Legumes and Beans – good carbs can help lower body weight without planned calorie restriction

- Anything high in protein – helpful in keeping your energy levels up in your efforts as a whole, even when you're in a period of fasting

- Anything with the herbs cayenne pepper, psyllium, or dried/crushed dandelion – they'll contribute to weight loss without sacrificing calories or effort

- Avocado – a high-, good-calorie fruit that has a lot of healthy fats

- Berries – often high in antioxidants and vitamin C as well as flavonoids for weight loss

- Cruciferous Vegetables – broccoli, cauliflower, brussel sprouts, and more are incredibly high in fiber, which you'll definitely want to keep constipation at bay with IF

- Eggs – high in protein and great for building muscle during IF periods

- Nuts & Grains – sources of healthy fats and essential fiber

- Potatoes – when prepared in healthy ways, they satiate hunger well and help with weight loss

- Wild-Caught Fish – high in healthy fats while providing protein and vitamin D for your brain

When it comes to liquids, some of it is pretty self-explanatory:

- Water:

- It's always good for you! It will help keep you hydrated, it will provide relief with headaches or lightheadedness or fatigue, and it clears out your system in the initial detox period.

- Try adding a squeeze of lemon, some cucumber or strawberry slices, or a couple of sprigs of mint, lavender, or basil to give your water some flavor if you're not enthused with the taste of it plain.

- If you need something other than water to drink, you can always seek out:

- Probiotic drinks like kefir or kombucha

- You can even look for probiotic foods such as sauerkraut, kimchi, miso, pickles, yogurt, tempeh, and more!

- Probiotics work amazingly well at healing your gut especially in times of intense transition, as with the start of intermittent fasting.

- Black coffee

- Sweeteners and milk aren't productive for your fasting and weight loss goals.

- Try black coffee whenever possible, in moderation.

- Heated or chilled vegetable or bone broths

- Teas of any kind

- Apple cider vinegar shots

- Instead, try water or other drinks with ACV mixed in.

Drinks to avoid would be:

- Regular soda

- Diet soda

- Alcohol of any kind

- Anything with artificial sweetener

- Artificial sweetener will shock your insulin levels into imbalance with your blood sugar later on.

Chapter 8: Frequency of Fasting

There are a lot of misconceptions that are associated with this diet, and in this section we'll bust the myths.

Skipping breakfast will make you gain weight

Breakfast might be considered to be the most important meal of the day, but it isn't, and that notion is nothing more than a myth. People believe that skipping breakfast leads to excessive hunger and weight gain. No scientific studies or research supports this claim. Skipping breakfast won't make you fat and you can do so quite safely without any fear.

Your metabolism improves when you eat frequently

It is a popular myth that eating frequently helps to improve your metabolism. Eating small meals does not improve your body's ability to burn calories. Yes, your body does need some energy to digest and assimilate the food you consume. It is referred to as the thermic effect of food, and it accounts for about 20-30% of total calories from protein, 5-10% from carbs and about 3% from fats. On an average, the thermic effect of food accounts for 10% of the total calories you consume. Take into consideration the total calories you consume and not the number of meals you eat. You don't have to keep eating regularly.

Eating frequently helps to keep hunger at bay

People believe that snacking continually helps to keep hunger at bay and reduces the chances of excessive hunger. Frequent meals will naturally leave you feeling full, but you don't have to do this. If you want to cut your cravings and keep hunger at bay, then you'll want to make sure that you are filling yourself up with the right kind of food. Your meals should contain high amounts of fiber, protein, and healthy fats instead of carbs. A meal that's rich in carbs will make you feel hungry soon and make you want to eat more food. Consuming carbs can make you crave more carbs. So, a balanced meal is the key to reducing your hunger.

Small meals assist in weight loss

Small meals won't do your body any good, and they certainly don't aid in weight loss. If you are worried that fasting leads to weight gain, you can lay those fears to rest.

The brain needs glucose

Yes, the brain needs glucose in order to function. It doesn't mean that you need to keep consuming carbs every couple of hours for your brain to continue working. It certainly won't stop performing if you don't eat anything for an extended period. This misconception is due to the assumption that the brain needs glucose for functioning. Your body starts producing glucose by a process known as gluconeogenesis. There is a reserve of glucose in the body, and your liver breaks this down to supply glucose that is essential for the functioning of your brain.

Eating often is necessary for proper health

Being in a fed state continuously isn't natural for the human body. During evolution, humans had to endure periods of starvation. If frequent meals were essential for survival, then the human race would have been wiped out a long time ago. In fact, fasting helps to induce cellular repair by kick starting the process of autophagy. It helps to protect against diseases like Alzheimer's and even certain types of cancers. Fasting is quite beneficial for the system, and it helps to cleanse the system by eliminating the build-up of toxins in the body. Snacking often has certain disadvantages. Frequent meals can easily increase your calorie intake and lead to a build-up of fatty cells in the liver.

Fasting shifts your body into "starvation mode"

A favorite argument against intermittent fasting is that it puts your body in starvation mode. While fasting, the body assumes that it's starving, and therefore shuts down its metabolism and prevents the burning of fat to produce energy. Long-term weight loss reduces the calories you burn, and that's what starvation mode is. However, this is bound to happen regardless of the dieting protocol you follow. Short-term fasting helps to speed up the metabolic function of the body. The increase in the levels of noradrenaline in the body increases the breaking down of the fat cells and thereby boosts the metabolism as well. Fasting for up to 48 hours helps to boost the metabolism, but anything more reverses this effect. You can fast as long as you follow a sensible fasting protocol.

You will lose muscle while fasting

Once again, it is nothing more than a misconception that fasting leads to muscle loss. Fasting leads to fat loss! In fact, intermittent fasting helps to increase the build-up of lean muscle and, when coupled with the right exercises, it helps to build muscle.

Chapter 9: Cleaning your body from toxins with intermittent fasting

Toxins that accumulate in the fatty tissue within the flesh are flushed out along with the fat that is burned; the mind realigns to what millions of years of nature's evolution has endowed it with; and the burden of an imbalanced existence is cast off in exchange for the energy and calm of the wise.

The human body is built in such a way that, when we eat, the nutrients are stored for future use to burn and create energy. This energy is in the form of fats and glycogen or sugars and carbs. Unfortunately, unlike our ancient ancestors, we are not eating everything in sight, so there is enough energy stored during seasons when food is scarce. Therefore, there are times our bodies are storing excess fats and glycogen that can cause issues. At that point, it is important to consider fasting or detoxing to get this stored energy out of our systems.

There are only two things we do as humans – we eat to store calories, or we fast to burn calories!

Fasting is actually the easiest and best way to maintain our body balance in regard to cleansing our bodies. Studies have shown that most people spend up to 20 hrs. eating! That means, when you constantly eat, whether meals or snacks, you are not burning anything. This, in turn, leads to a problem with not being able to lose weight and, in fact, putting weight on.

What's alarming, when you constantly eat, you are giving your body more calories than it can process. The only way you can restore your body to a healthy balance is to stop overeating and incorporate a detox that will clean out these unwanted calories and literally clean out your body, so it can function properly.

Unfortunately, our society turns an evil eye to people who are detoxing and cleansing their bodies, claiming they are harming themselves. In reality, they are cleansing their bodies and getting themselves in a better place. Keep in mind, the food industry is up in arms that anyone would step back on constant eating and eat less because it's bad for business.

More people are starting to realize their eating habits are killing them. They are more aware that it is up to them to take better care of their health and turn away from the food industry that is shoving processed foods onto people. Welcome the nutritional industry that is gaining popularity for people to help them understand the value of good nutrition and how to make sure they are doing the right thing for their own health. Unfortunately, there are a million nutritional programs that claim they have "proof" about their chosen programs. Eat six small meals a day and lose weight! Live on weight loss shakes that have their own issues, eat protein bars or cereal, and once again, just continue to overeat and see how well that goes for you.

Step by step instructions to do kidney detox with fasting

Kidney purifying fasts, also called kidney detoxification, are utilized to enhance kidney work and keep away from kidney stones. So as to choose if kidney detoxification is advantageous, you should first know its impacts on the body.

Understand the capacity of the kidneys and urinary framework. The normal individual is conceived with 2 kidneys. They are a part of your body's urinary framework, alongside the ureters and the bladder. The kidneys have various capacities, including adjusting body liquids, adjusting body chemicals, expelling waste items and discharging fundamental hormones. They are basic to your different organs since they process and expel the collection of waste items, including chemicals, salt and surplus water. The following work will break down how the components of a kidney purging fast influence the body.

Counsel your specialist before beginning a kidney purifying quick.

A few people are in danger for kidney malady. On the off chance that anybody in your family has had kidney infection, it is a smart thought to get circulatory strain, blood and pee tests to decide your general kidney wellbeing.

A kidney purifying fast may likewise restrain medicine ingestion.

Lessen the measure of food you gobble in the days prior to your fast.

Fasting frequently builds sentiments of appetite. This early decrease in eating routine can check your appetite.

For a few people this might be the main advance required; making a sound eating routine and expanding your liquid admission might be sufficient to scrub the kidneys.

Numerous kidney sickness patients are advised to restrict their admission from food that is high in protein, cholesterol and sodium. The kidneys are in charge of preparing these substances, and this adjustment in eating routine can permit the kidneys to rest some time, during or after the wash down.

Figure out what your liquid consumption ought to be. Most kidney purifying fasts last around 3 days and they suggest that you devour half of your body weight in ounces. For instance on the off chance that you weigh 180 lbs. (81.6 kg), you should drink 90 oz. (2.66 l) of water every day.

Liquids are fundamental to a kidney purging fast because your kidneys channel and clean around 200 qt. (189.27 l) of liquid from your blood each day. Around 198 qt. (187.377 l) are assimilated and 2 qt. (1.89 l) proceed to the bladder to form urine.

Many purging fasts prescribe the use of refined water since it doesn't have the mineral substance of tap water. This likewise permits your kidneys to rest by constraining the quantity of minerals your kidneys should process.

Receive a fluid eating regimen for 3 days that incorporates water, juice, natural teas and vegetable juices. Stay away from liquor, caffeine and dairy items.

Fluids help to rehydrate the body, which is fundamental to averting kidney stones, which are crystalline stones that form when a man is got dried out and a lot of a substance, similar to calcium, is in the urine.

Teas produced using celery seeds or vexes go about as normal diuretics. Parsley and bearberry are normally utilized as a part of teas as they help the stomach related and urinary system.

Liquor, caffeine and milk products are diuretics, which make you urinate all the more regularly and dispose of liquids rapidly, in this way getting dried out the body before essential liquids are absorbed.

Vegetable stock is made by steaming vegetables or vegetable peels, including carrots, celery and beets for 60 minutes, and afterward stressing and drinking the supplement rich liquid. Drink this stock 2 to 3 times each day to battle electrolyte and potassium problem.

Eat watermelon to rinse kidneys after your 3 day quick.

Watermelon is a characteristic diuretic, however not at all like liquor and caffeine; it doesn't appear to strain the kidneys. A watermelon wash down encourages the liver to process amonia, a loss from protein assimilation, and convey it to the urea. This likewise facilitates strain on the kidneys, while freeing the collection of surplus liquids.

There are numerous approaches to get this advantage from watermelon. It can be cut up and eaten entire (with seeds) or squeezed. The seeds can be made into tea, and the tissue can be made into soup.

Back yourself gradually out of the fast by eating crude vegetables.

Any adjustment in diet ought to be gradually adopted to maintain a strategic distance from discombobulating, sickness or appetite problem. In the wake of eating vegetables for a couple of days, fuse little measures of protein, and after that move again into a typical, solid eating regimen.

Chapter 10: The Biggest Mistakes to Avoid

Continuing to Eat Crap Food

One of the most common complaints people make is that they are following the fasting technique but aren't seeing results. When asked about their nutrition, the answer always reveals the problem. They are still eating processed foods (chips, candy, cake, crackers, etc.) and drinking sweetened beverages (sweet teas and soda). You cannot fast, exercise hard, eat junk food, and still expect that you will lose fat and tone that butt. You must decide to throw away all the unhealthy stuff and go for whole and unprocessed foods. There will be cheat days when you can indulge in something decadent, but don't make that part of your intermittent fasting lifestyle.

Not Eating Enough in the Feeding Period

Not getting enough to eat after a fast is a common mistake. The stomach has a certain amount of dispensability. Meaning it can shrink and expand to a certain amount. While in a fast, it contracts and adapts to handling less. When you are eating a lot, it expands and gets used to accommodate larger amounts of food. When you are preparing to break your fast, you naturally want to eat heavy foods that are very dense.

Coffee and Tea Creamers

This is another common mistake that people unintentionally do that causes a break in fast without realizing it. Even a half-tablespoon of coffee creamer or almond milk is enough to trigger an insulin response and break a fast. As soon as you include the substance in your beverage, you may as well end the fast because you will need to start over. Adjusting to coffee in black can be difficult if it is not what you are accustomed to. Many people that cannot seem to get used to it simply switch to herbal teas.

Not Drinking Enough Water

Another common mistake is simply not keeping yourself hydrated enough. Many times, when you feel like you may be hungry, it may actually be your body telling you to hydrate it. Women were shocked to find that many hunger pains during a fast were curbed by simply drinking water or tea. The body also demands more salt on an intermittent fasting diet. Be sure to get enough water and salt as these are essential to getting good, healthy results. Drinking enough water and staying well hydrated also helps to prevent and get over the keto flu, if you are also following the ketogenic diet. Hydration is key to any change in diet and will nearly always improve your results.

Not Having Enough Support

Often times with any diet this is the biggest cause of failure. Support for a life change is absolutely a necessity. Without having a support system to lean on, ask questions and discuss ideas with, most people are not successful. If you are struggling and frustrated, be sure to find someone who is also going through the changes and adjustments that come with changing your habits to an intermittent fasting lifestyle. There are many online support groups with great support systems and knowledge to share. Changing your life is hard as it is and it is nearly impossible to do alone.

Not Keeping Yourself Busy

You cannot spend the day fasting and sitting around doing nothing. Staying idle is the worst thing you can do because you will start thinking about food. Get up and do something to stay active, as long as it keeps you away from food.

You Set Goals Too High

If you are a newbie to intermittent fasting, make sure that you don't start off with only one meal a day. You may think that going in hard from the start will help you torch all that fat, but it doesn't work that way. You cannot go from eating four to six meals a day to surviving on a single meal.

You Fear Going Hungry

It's perfectly normal to feel hungry, but you will not die just because you go for a couple of hours without food. Most people have this irrational and morbid fear of depriving themselves of food, believing that all their muscles will be gobbled up. This fear can tempt you to cheat during your fasting window. Do not be afraid of a bit of hunger.

You Spend Your Days Staring at the Clock

Most newbies will develop an obsession with the clock when fasting. They will count down the hours, minutes, and seconds until they can rush to the kitchen and start bingeing. On the other extreme end are people who are afraid of breaking the "rules," so they make sure that they fast until the last second of the fasting window is over. Intermittent fasting is not that hard or strict. You cannot spend the day worrying and wondering about the timeframes and schedules. If your entire life starts and ends with your next meal, you will drive yourself mad. Just relax and enjoy the ride.

Obsessing Over the Sum of the Parts

Intermittent fasting is like a complex and dynamic system. There are a lot of individual pieces that form a large system. It is useless getting fixated on one small piece and forgetting that there are many more important things to focus on. For example, some people may worry about whether adding a teaspoon of cream to their coffee while fasting will ruin their chances of losing fat.

Chapter 11: How to Get the Best Out of Intermittent Fasting

Combining Intermittent Fasting with Exercise

There are many ways to exercise including cardio, strength training or lifting, yoga, and Pilates. Any of these exercise styles and regiments can be beneficial and help with your ultimate goal of weight loss and a healthier life, but certain workouts have certain benefits. There are also time frames to exercise in during a fast that will help to optimize your results. Cardio is ideal for fat burning and strength training for building muscle. Yoga is great for core strength and certain yoga poses can actually help to regulate certain hormones. Nearly all exercise has benefits if you can find the time and the drive to make it part of your daily lifestyle.

When to Work Out

Most would consider the opportune time to work out to be in the middle of a fast. For example, let's say you started your fast at ten at night, working out after you wake up in the morning is considering an ideal time to work out or exercise as it is in the middle of your fast. You should still have ample energy as your body will not be expecting to be fed until later. Working out in the morning is also a great way to get going in the morning and is a natural way of waking up. Doing your work out in the middle or beginning of your fast is usually superior and you will feel better with better results as opposed to doing your work out toward the end of your fast.

Yoga and Pilates to Aid in Hormonal Balance

Many people have heard of the wonderful benefits of practicing yoga and Pilates. Yoga is relaxing, great for flexibility, and improving core and body strength. Yoga has been known to aid in pain relief and improve the mood, reset the mind and help with focus. Yoga is a great natural way to give your body a boost and to help relax and de-stress. Basically, yoga brings the three main elements together; exercise, breathing, and meditation. Pilates has a similar effect except it tends to focus more on lengthening and strengthening all the major and large muscle groups. Pilates particularly improves strength, body awareness, and balance. What is less known about Pilates and yoga is that it can actually help to stabilize and regulate the body's hormones with certain poses. The yoga poses can subtly pressurize and depressurize certain glands of the body.

These minor compressions and decompressions can help to regulate hormonal secretions. Therefore, certain yoga poses can help to balance and stimulate certain endocrine functions. Many common negative feelings can be attributed to a hormonal imbalance. Feelings like being constantly tired, low self-esteem, anxiety, and emotional eating with a slow metabolism can all possible be effects of a hormonal imbalance in women.

Cardio — Running, Cycling, and Swimming to Help with Intermittent Fasting Results

There was a myth going around for a while that doing cardio on an empty stomach can help with losing the 'stubborn' fat. This is false. Doing fasted cardio is actually what helps to lose those stubborn fat places. To define what exactly cardiovascular exercise is, it is an aerobic exercise that uses oxygen to meet the demands of energy during exercising. Examples of cardio workouts are swimming, running, cycling — basically any aerobic type activity. This basically means it is an exercise that specifically works the heart, the lungs, and that oxygen intake is required to participate in.

Strength Training and Intermittent Fasting

Strength training combined with intermittent fasting and healthy eating can provide some truly great results. Strength training, also known as weight lifting or resistance training is anaerobic exercise based off using resistance to cause muscle contraction, which in turn builds muscle, improves anaerobic endurance and enlarges the size of the skeletal muscles.

Meditation and Mindfulness

Meditation can be an excellent tool for focus, clearing the mind and aiding in success with any lifestyle change, especially intermittent fasting. It is an ancient technique that helps to focus and clear the mind. Meditation actually changes the structure of the brain and allows it to be clear and promote simple clear thoughts. It can give you almost superhuman abilities like being able to keep a calm clear head in a high-pressure situation and use the power of the mind to your advantage.

Chapter 12: Combining Intermittent Fasting with Other Diets

Since intermittent fasting is not really a diet, it is a pattern of feeding and fasting, and many women combine it with other diet plans. Intermittent fasting goes along great with other diets and women are getting great results. Intermittent fasting is compatible with many diets because it is adjustable and based less off of what is being consumed and more of when food is being consumed. The most popular diets that intermittent fasting is combined with is the ketogenic diet, the gluten-free diet, the paleo diet, and a vegan diet.

Combining Intermittent Fasting with a Ketogenic Diet

Combining both a keto diet and an intermittent fasting lifestyle is probably the best, quickest, and most effective way to lose weight. The keto diet is incredibly popular because it is so effective, especially in women.

The keto diet is based on high fat because fat is one of the first sources of fuel that your body converts into energy when consumed. By feeding your body high in healthy fat foods, it helps it to be more efficient in the breakdown. There are numerous benefits to combining intermittent fasting with a ketogenic diet; you will get very few cravings for starters. One of the desirable effects of the ketogenic diet is that it is exceptional at stabilizing blood sugar. Since keto is fat based, you will not get spikes in your blood sugar and therefore your insulin will not rise and give you food cravings. A ketogenic diet already is known for suppressing hunger. When you are on a ketogenic diet, it encourages the liver to produce more keynotes. The ketones get into your bloodstream and the cells use them as fuel. Ketones also are known for suppressing ghrelin, the body's hormone that tells you when to eat. With the ketogenic diet already suppressing your hunger, fasting comes significantly easier and allows you to fast in longer windows and get the benefits of a longer fast.

Combining Intermittent Fasting with a Vegan Diet

Combining intermittent fasting with a vegan diet can be a greater challenge as vegan or plant-based food does not have healthy fats as readily available as animal-based foods. Having said that, it is not impossible and can still be conducive with the lifestyle of intermittent fasting. Basically, the difference between eating a regular diet and eating a vegan diet is that vegans do not eat any animal-based foods. They strictly eat plant-based foods and fruits, vegetables and substitutes like tofu etc. What makes combining veganism with intermittent fasting difficult the lack of natural fats available. When your body enters a fat burning state, it is more difficult to break a fast without any animal-based product. It is not impossible though and many vegans have had luck with it. Like with any diet, there are loopholes and ways to make it work with your lifestyle. Many vegans simply just have to eat more carbs. Nuts and seeds are good sources of protein and fat and are popular in a vegan diet in general.

Combining with a Paleo Diet

Combining intermittent fasting with a paleo diet is about as simple as you can get. Basically, a paleo diet is a diet based off what food was consumed during the stone ages and ancient times. When there were no stores, supermarkets, delis, and fast food restaurants, what was left? There were plants, meats, berries, vegetables, and whatever food could be hunted, picked, made or gathered.

The Gluten-Free Diet and Intermittent Fasting

Many people have seen the effects and benefits of going gluten-free. People with digestive and stomach issues often change to gluten-free. Gluten-free goes just as well with intermittent fasting as any other diet. It is important to keep an eye on your caloric intake as gluten-free diets often are carb free as well. Gluten-free diets tend to have a lot of foods that contain a lot of flour, so watch out for the carb count when eating gluten-free. Many women that are gluten-free already have good grasps of what goes well with their diet and where they can find foods that work for them. Adding in the timed fasting is just one step further that can take you closer to your goals and help to lead to a better and healthier life.

Chapter 13: Essential Oils to Help with Intermittent Fasting and Weight Loss

Essential oils are a rapidly growing fad and are useful for many different ailments and can provide support for multiple body systems. While the use of essential oils is controversial in their effectiveness, many women swear by them and there is some evidence they can help with weight loss as well as provide immune support as well as mental health support. The route in which to use essential oils is varied. They can be used in a diffuser, inhaled in an inhaler, rubbed on the skin, made into body wraps, burned in candles, and many more options. They work both topically and aromatically. There are five specific essential oils geared toward weight loss as well as many that help with psychological challenges.

Grapefruit Essential Oils

Grapefruit essential oils contain d-limonene, a chemical that increases the rate of the metabolism because it induces lipolysis or the breakdown of fat cells. Grapefruit essential oils also help to fight cellulite in women. Grapefruit essential oils work best as a massage oil or bath salt. Grapefruit essential oils can be used daily for best results.

Peppermint Essential Oils

Peppermint is a great oil for energy and can really help to stifle cravings. It is refreshing to smell and has positive effects when inhaled; it is a natural bronchodilator and helps improve oxygen flow. Peppermint essential oils work best when inhaled directly. Put it in a diffuser for twenty minutes a day or put several drops onto a cloth or handkerchief and inhale directly for best results.

Lemon Essential Oils

Lemon smells fantastic and is quite useful in helping to block out thoughts of greasy foods and sugar. It has properties that help to improve energy and helps to increase your mood. Lemon essential oils are great for right before a workout. It works best in a diffuser for fifteen to twenty minutes.

Rosemary Essential Oils

Rosemary has an herbal, refreshing type smell and can really help in suppressing the appetite. Rosemary can help with water retention and surpass craving as well as help with cellulite prevention. Give it a sniff when you are struggling with a certain food craving. It is also a great massage oil and is effective as a bath salt. Rosemary has other health benefits as well and can even help with menstrual-related bloating.

Ginger Essential Oils

Ginger is a powerful detox aid. Ginger has detoxifying effects that are quite helpful with purging the body and mind of cravings and toxins. Ginger also helps to stimulate the lymph nodes, and it helps to stimulate blood flow and goes great in a bath! Many women mix with coconut oil and use topically. Ginger should be used with some caution as it is a "hot" oil and can cause the feelings of burning. Mixing four to five drops of ginger essential oil and two to three tablespoons of coconut oil and adding it to your bath is a great way to reap the benefits of ginger!

Lavender Essential Oils

Lavender is perhaps the most popular and well-known essential oil. Probably because it has such a diverse range of uses and effects. Lavender's best known for its calming properties. These are especially useful for when and if you experience 'hanger' or anxiety during a fast. Lavender helps to calm the irritability. Lavender is also a good sleep aid and can be used in a variety of forms. It can be applied topically, inhaled or ingested.

While essential oils certainly are not for everyone, they can and do help many women to overcome struggles both with intermittent fasting and wit weight loss in general. Sometimes, a sniff of the right oil is all you need to get over the hurdle at hand, whether it is to maintain a fast or get past a craving. The first few days of a fast or diet are always the most difficult and any support you can get is usually worth considering. They certainly have a place in a healthy life if you are willing to give them a try.

Chapter 14: Supplements and Vitamins to Aid in Fasting

Getting adequate vitamins and proper nutrition is absolutely vital while doing the intermittent fasting lifestyle. It is especially important because intermittent fasting is essentially forcing your body into a state of fat burning. In a state of fat burning, you are also in ketosis typically. Taking supplemental vitamins may be necessary during your fasting periods, especially if you are engaging in a long-term fast. Most multivitamins will due, but it is important to know what is in them and what they should contain to aid with your fast.

Sodium and Potassium

Levels of ketones in the bloodstream rise during your periods of fasting which cause your body to signal a flushing response. This quickly depletes the stores of potassium and sodium. It can cause fatigue, low energy, and the feeling of being lightheaded. These minerals are very important for ketogenesis and without them, the body really must work and struggle to access the stores of fat.

Magnesium

Magnesium is a body mineral that regulates several vital body functions. Magnesium helps to regulate nerve and blood pressure and is easily and swiftly depleted in the period of fasting. Low magnesium is what can cause the feeling of brain fogginess or muscle cramps during a fasting period.

B-Complex Vitamins

B-complex vitamin, which includes riboflavin, niacin, thiamine, and biotin are vitamins that aid the body in absorbing nutrients. B-complex vitamins do not get flushed out of the body in the same way sodium, potassium, and magnesium does during the state of ketosis. However, there are a large number of women that are chronically low or have B-complex vitamin deficiencies.

Vitamin D

Vitamin D is a very common deficiency amongst both men and women. Vitamin D is rather difficult to obtain through food intake and is acquired naturally through sunlight. Vitamin D is vital to both immune health and bone density. Vitamin D helps the use nutrients that are critical to body functions and helps allow the nutrients to function, magnesium being one of them.

Chromium

Chromium is not as common in your everyday multivitamin but there has been some research that shows it can be a culprit that mitigates hunger. This can be problematic as it may force you to end your fast earlier than planned or expected due to the hunger pangs.

Beta-Hydroxybutyrate or BHB

Many women who intermittently fast also take a BHB supplement as well, these are also known as exogenous ketones. This means ketones that are not produced by the body. One of the three ketone bodies is BHB. Ketone bodies are what is naturally produced by the liver when you are in a state of ketosis. If broken down to the cellular level, the human body needs BHB to access and adequately use the fat stores for energy. Using a BHB supplement during a fast helps to ensure that the body will have the necessary levels of BHB in the bloodstream. Having the proper levels of BHB in the bloodstream will help to facilitate the metabolizing of fat into energy.

Water (H2O)

Drinking water is absolutely vital to any and all diets and fasts. This cannot be stressed enough. Lack of hydration is often the biggest factor in nearly all negative side effects to any fast. Body organs and tissues including the brain depend and utilize water to maintain the proper levels of nutrients, vitamins, and minerals. Dehydration has a wide variety of symptoms and can quickly lead to fatigue, irritability, dizziness, confusion, headache, and many other symptoms and feelings of discomfort. Maintaining proper hydration throughout a fast is important and allows any supplemental vitamins to work better.

Chapter 15: When Women Should Avoid Intermittent Fasting

While intermittent fasting is flexible, versatile, and adaptable to many different lifestyles, it is still the case that many women should probably *not* attempt IF, for the sake of their overall health.

However, even with these limitations in place, there is lingering potential for each of these types of women to come to a place of progress or healing eventually that would allow them to move through their struggles and attempt IF at their own pace. Therefore, if you qualify as any of the following candidates, don't be too dejected or hopeless! With the appropriate personal growth and the right lessons being presented to you, you'll surely come back to intermittent fasting as soon as you're ready for it.

Pregnant

You are pregnant - This is because pregnant women have a higher demand for more energy and nutrients that come from what they eat and drink. But really, some women should not even try experimenting with intermittent fasting at all. If you do not feast or fast properly, you risk become infertile or early onset menopause: even if you are in your twenties.

You having a history of any kind of eating disorder – Individuals who have suffered from an eating disorder are more likely to develop another eating disorder at some point in their lives. Fasting and feasting could lead patients with unhealthy eating patterns to develop additional problems.

You are chronically stressed or do not handle physical or mental stress well – people who experience constant chronic stress should not limit their diet or meals because they may actually need more nourishment.

You have insomnia or unusual sleeping habits – Just like individuals with chronic stress, if you have trouble sleeping, then you need to be nurturing your body not adding more stress.

If you are new to exercising and dieting and this is the first time you are trying a new lifestyle.

Now that you fully understand the science behind fasting, as well as the many benefits and myths behind the method, you are now prepared to read all about the different types of intermittent fasting plans. Everyone has their own needs when it comes to incorporating a new lifestyle; Jill may work a full time job and have a family to take care of, while Katie is a full time student who works out five days a week. Whatever your needs are, there is a way to adopt intermittent fasting without it disrupting your everyday life.

Although intermittent fasting can give you increased energy, better metabolism, and stronger cellular protection, the risks clearly outweigh the benefits for pregnant IF candidates. Since the female body is made to bear children, the effects of intermittent fasting are already debated in their relation to female health, but when it comes to pregnant and soon-to-be mothers, the answer to the question is a clear "No." Pregnant women should not be working with intermittent fasting.

For the expecting mother, long periods between meals are not necessarily such a good thing. The pregnant woman will need to be eating whenever she's hungry to gain the weight and nutrients her future child will need to survive. Furthermore, she will need to combat the morning sickness and nausea that go along with pregnancy, and if she's concerned about her timing with the intermittent fast, she might put herself in a detrimental situation for her overall health by mistake.

If you're recently pregnant but had used intermittent fasting previously with great success, you can shift back to focusing on *what* you eat rather than *when* you eat. Just as it is for the standard person shifting from normal eating to intermittent fasting and going from *what*'s eaten to *when* it's eaten, when you switch from IF to pregnancy, you'll shift eating habits once again. This time, however, you'll try to make sure you're eating the best foods whenever possible; not just in your okayed eating windows.

If you're having trouble stopping your intermittent fast while you've just become pregnant, you might want to reconsider the reasons behind your IF in the first place. Is it really for your health, or does it support your controlling tendency to limit your weight? Try to make sure that when you're pregnant, you're looking for what supports your health, rather than your mental image of what you should look like and what you think you should weigh. Pregnancy is a beautiful time, but it's not about restriction, it's about abundance and weight gain and growth, so it doesn't mesh well with IF at all.

Underweight

For women who are already underweight, intermittent fasting might not be the best thing for your health. Surely, there are unintentionally underweight women who don't have the time they'd like to have for eating or who don't have the energy they'd like to have for cooking, but there are also intentionally underweight women who are looking for an additional method to use to keep off that "excess" weight for good.

If you're incredibly underweight already (even if you don't feel like it!), steer clear of intermittent fasting. If you're only five to ten pounds underweight and you're seeking spiritual enlightenment, lessened brain fog, or a jolt to your digestive system, IF may work just fine for you without being problematic. (While you *might* find a method of IF that works alright for you in this case, don't make the hard and fast decisions on eating pattern switching without first making sure to consult a doctor or health professional.)

Eating Disorder

For the individual with an eating disorder, no matter what variety, intermittent fasting may seem to be helpful, but it will only function as a trigger for that person's disorder. No matter who you are, if you approach intermittent fasting for healing or weight loss, you're probably doing so because you want to switch from stuffing yourself of emptiness to healing yourself with goodness. Your focus, in other words, likely falls on growth (not physically but emotionally, spiritually, mentally, and regarding health capacity) rather than withering.

For the individual suffering from an eating disorder, all attempts toward health and growth are skewed by distortions of body image and self-esteem. Essentially, all attempts toward health and growth are twisted by the compulsory drive to purge. If you or someone you know struggled or struggles with anorexia, bulimia, orthorexia, binge eating, purging, avoidant/restrictive food intake disorder, or any other eating disorder, be extremely curious and demanding with them if they share an interest in intermittent fasting.

Question their inspirations and drives; demand they are honest with you. The likelihood is greater than not that this person is using intermittent fasting as a way to lose weight they can't afford to lose rather than to get healthier in general. If you're able to discern it at all, the individual's reason for *starting* IF is the best way to ascertain their true intentions. It can be hard to tell who has an eating disorder and who doesn't, but the way people talk about food, body image, fasting, and dieting can reveal more than you could ever anticipate. And once you *can* tell who has an eating disorder, help them stay clear from IF because it can really exacerbate their circumstances despite their (and your) best intentions.

Diabetic

If you're already on insulin, as a diabetic most likely, you're already working to keep your levels of blood sugar at balance. If you add into the mix IF work to increase or decrease insulin resistance (to help with weight loss), you'll put yourself in a truly dangerous spot. People with diabetes should absolutely *not* skip doses of insulin to lose weight by lowering blood sugar. This would be disastrous for someone who has diabetes because they'd surely lose the weight, but they'd feel drained to a disastrous degree because humans do *need* this sugar or glucose in our blood to derive energy.

So, if you have diabetes, stay away from intermittent fasting. As with the pregnant candidate, you could try to switch the foods you're eating instead of when you're eating. By adding the right, healthful foods into your diet, you might find that the weight that sticks to you so stubbornly can be depleted with your condition being made none the worse. However, be careful if you're diabetic when it comes to *fasting disguised as dieting*. If you feel inclined to try a juice or liquid diet, second guess those inclinations, for it's very likely that this type of diet would cause extra stress to your system, what with the high glycemic and fiber-free contents of some juices.

Basically, if you're diabetic and feeling inclined to make your life healthier, don't limit *when* you eat and don't just drink liquids. Rather than restricting whatsoever, try to *incorporate* healthier, more whole foods that are oriented towards healing innately and then maybe add exercise into the mix when you're ready for it.

Chapter 16: Different Methods of Intermittent Fasting

While there are many methods for intermittent fasting, only a handful of them works well specifically for women, and others work well for women in special cases. Overall, the goal is to learn about each method, its strengths, and its weaknesses, and then to choose which is right for you, given the current stage of your life and what struggles you face at the moment.

Crescendo Method

The crescendo method of intermittent fasting is the one voted most productive for female-bodied practitioners. This method is well-known for its gentle approach to fasting, its caution, and awareness of hormonal balance, its ability to help you lose weight, and its gradual introduction (which works especially well for women with inconsistent work or life schedules).

Through the crescendo method, the individual will fast 12 to 16 hours at a time for two or three days a week that is not consecutive days. For instance, she might fast Sunday, normally eat Monday and Tuesday, fast Wednesday, normally eat Thursday, fast Friday, eat normally on Saturday, and repeat the pattern the next Sunday. During fast days, light cardio exercises or yoga can be practiced, but no intense workouts are allowed, due to the long hours involved in the fast. As needed, drink lots of water (with salt added if/when you get dizzy!) and coffee if you desire any energy boosts.

After two successful weeks of this pattern of fasting, additional days can be added, or the timing can be tweaked based on what's working and what isn't. These method amps up the power after the initial detoxification period, based on the abilities and reach of the individual. It builds in effect, but the impact remains the same such as increased health and decreased weight while respecting hormones and the potential for hefty mood swings.

Lean-Gains Method (14:10)

The lean-gains method has several different incarnations on the web, but its fame comes from the fact that it helps shed fat while building it into muscle almost immediately. Through the lean-gains method, you'll find yourself able to shift all that fat to be muscle through a rigorous practice of fasting, eating right, and exercising.

Through this method, you fast anywhere from 14 to 16 hours and then spend the remaining 10 or 8 hours each day engaged in eating and exercise. This method, as opposed to the crescendo, features daily fasting and eating, rather than alternated days of eating versus not. Therefore, you don't have to be quite so cautious about extending the physical effort to exercise on the days you are fasting because those days when you're fasting are literally every day!

For the lean-gains method, start fasting only 14 hours and work it up to 16 if you feel comfortable with it, but never forget to drink enough water and be careful about expending too much energy on exercise! Remember that you want to *grow* in health and potential through intermittent fasting. You'll certainly not want to lose any of that growth by forcing the process along.

20:4 Method

Stepping things up a notch from the 14:10 and 16:8 methods, the 20:4 method is a tough one to master, for it is rather unforgiving. People talk about this method of intermittent fasting as intense and highly restrictive, but they also say that the effects of living this method are almost unparalleled with all other tactics.

For the 20:4 method, you'll fast for 20 hours each day and squeeze all your meals, all your eating, and all your snacking into 4 hours. People who attempt 20:4 normally have two smaller meals or just one large meal and a few snacks during their 4-hour window to eat, and it really is up to the individual which four hours of the day they devote to eating.

The trick for this method is to make sure you're not overeating or bingeing during those 4-hour windows to eat. It is all-too-easy to get hungry during the 20-hour fast and have that feeling then propel you into intense and unrealistic hunger or meal sizes after the fast period is over. Be careful if you try this method. If you're new to intermittent fasting, work your way up to this one gradually, and if you're working your way up already, only make the shift to 20:4 when you know you're ready. It would surely disappoint if all your progress with intermittent fasting got hijacked by one poorly thought-out goal with 20:4 method.

16/8 Method

This method is also popularly known as the Leangains method. It is a short routine of intermittent fasting that will help you burn body fat and improve your lean muscle. In this diet, you should fast for 16 hours daily, and your eating window is restricted to 8 hours a day. For instance, you can start your fast at 7 p.m. and then fast until 11 a.m. the following day. So, you can break your fast with a meal at noon and end with a meal at night before 7 p.m. If you start your fast on Monday night, it will extend until noon on Tuesday and so on. You can move onto this method of fasting after your body gets used to the previous method of fasting. This variant of intermittent fasting is quite simple. It can be as simple as skipping your breakfast instead of having your first meal at noon.

Most of us tend to lead busy lives, and hardly any of us have the time to eat breakfast. Yes, it is as simple as that. Skip your breakfast, have a nutritious lunch, a snack, and end your day with a nutritious dinner. You shouldn't have any snacks post dinner and no more late-night snacks. It will also help regulate your circadian rhythm. If you have dinner at 7 or 8 at night, you can give your body sufficient time to digest the meal before you go to bed.

24-Hour Protocol

Also known as the Eat-Stop-Eat diet. As the name suggests, in this variation of intermittent fasting, you should fast for 24 hours at a stretch. However, you shouldn't fast more than twice a week. You can start with one day and then increase it to two days a week. As mentioned, you should never fast on two consecutive days. You can select your fasting window, and you should stick to it. You can start your fast at 8 p.m. and end it on 8 p.m. on the following day. You can fast on Monday and Wednesday. You'll need to fast for 24 hours in a day. Therefore, you will not have an eating window during this fast. While you fast, you can have plenty of calorie-free beverages. So you can have your coffee, but don't add any sugar, cream or milk to it. Herbal teas and water should be your go-to drinks. If you want, you can even spruce up your regular drinking water by adding a couple of slices of lemon and sprigs of mint.

12:12 Method

As another of the easier methods of intermittent fasting, 12:12 method is well-suited to beginning practitioners. Many people actually live out 12:12 method without any forethought simply because of their sleeping and eating schedule but turning 12:12 into a conscious practice can have just as many positive effects on your life as the more drastic 20:4 method claims.

Alternate Fasting

Alternate day fasting, or the "every other day diet," is fairly self-explanatory. Eat for one full day, fast for one full day, repeat. This does not mean to fast from the moment you wake up until the end of the day but eat three square meals the next day. When practicing alternate day fasting, you should eat at least one meal every day. This may mean eating breakfast before 9 o'clock in the morning then abstaining from food until the same time the next day, or it could involve eating dinner by 7 o'clock in the evening and abstaining until 7 o'clock the following evening. Whatever time works best for you can be the beginning or ending time of your 24-hour fasting and feeding windows. This diet drastically reduces the calorie intake over the whole week because you are removing multiple days' worth of calories from the equation. Fasting for a full day between feast days allows the body to spend more time in a fat burning unfed state. On feasting days, you can eat whatever you'd like. For optimal weight loss, sticking to a healthy diet and not bingeing with carbs or unhealthy snacks is ideal. Some people practice this method with the same caloric restrictions as the 5:2 diet, so on fasting days, they are allowed 500 to 600 calories. Some studies have shown that this level of calorie intake is easier to maintain than full fasts and overall it is similar in effectiveness.

The "every other day" method has not proven to be any more effective than utilizing a diet that involves daily calorie restriction, but some people find it easier to restrict every other day so they can still enjoy an unrestricted diet half of the time. Both will yield similar fat loss results, but the intermittent fasting method has shown more successful in preserving muscle mass. This muscle mass is crucial to the burning of calories. It has also been shown that, in some cases, following this method can cause the body to feel less hungry during restricted periods than it would on a standard, calorie restrictive diet and can decrease the likelihood of binge eating on feast days.

Hormones such as ghrelin that cause the body to feel hungry when it is fasting can decrease, and the hormones that cause it to feel satiated increases. The concern with this diet is that intermittent fasting is not always a permanent lifestyle choice and a diet like this can increase the likelihood of bingeing later on. When you are used to a full binge one day and a full restriction the next, you can lose touch with what true hunger or satiety feels like. When you resume consuming food on a daily basis, the eating habits you may have become accustomed to bingeing and may lead to weight gain.

This method is also not ideal for women. The female body reacts differently than the male body to extended periods of fasting. A full 24 hours of fasting is riskier for women, but still within the allowed time frame. Extended fasts in women can change hormone levels drastically and over time can cause permanent damage to the reproductive system, possibly even leading to infertility. If you are a woman who would like to utilize this type of eating schedule, it is possible, but it's important to understand the risks associated with it. It is also important to avoid implementing such a long period of food avoidance if your body is not already accustomed to fasting. Start by fasting for 12 hours, then gradually increase the fasting window until you reach 24 hours to avoid a major shock to the body that can cause hormonal imbalances with potentially dangerous side effects.

Eat-Stop-Eat Diet

If you do not want to fast quite as consistently, try incorporating a 24-hour fast into your diet once or twice a week. This method is called the "eat - stop - eat" diet. The 24 hour fasting period should be scheduled so that you are consuming some form of sustenance every day. For instance, let's say you eat breakfast at 8:30 in the morning on Tuesday morning. You finish eating by 9 o'clock and begin your fast. At 9 o'clock in the morning on Wednesday morning, you can break your fast. Incorporating this type of fasting into your lifestyle once or twice a week can allow the same type of caloric deficit as other methods while not interfering as much with normal day-to-day activities. This method may be ideal if you like to do heavy workouts on many days of the week. Incorporating fasting on your rest days can allow you to fuel yourself well on work days and decrease consumption on days when you are burning fewer calories. In the same form as other methods, sticking to healthier foods on feast days can help to achieve the results while also avoiding feelings of weakness and lethargy during the fasting period.

The eat - stop - eat method will be helpful in reaching a caloric deficit and losing weight. However, this method may not yield the same caliber of results as others because the fasting is less consistent. The body will remain more accustomed to being in a fed state and therefore not gain quite the same level of benefits as more frequent fasting. It is still an effective method and will still be beneficial to the body's processes. Eat - stop - eat may be a good option for you if you are new to fasting or if you find it difficult to add a fasting schedule into your busy life.

Some people extend their fast little by little until it lasts for a duration of multiple days to increase the amount of time the body is in a fat burning state. Long-term fasting has been shown to dramatically increase levels of the human growth hormone and noradrenaline. These two hormones are essential to fat burning, muscle growth, muscle preservation, energy levels, mental clarity, cellular repair, and anti-aging. Extended fasting also allows the body to enter and remain in a state of ketosis which will burn more stored fat and increase the rapidity of weight loss. It is wise to consult a doctor before incorporating long fasting periods into your lifestyle. For women, fasting for more than 24 hours at a time can have adverse effects on hormone levels and may cause permanent damage to the body. It may also not be smart if you have health problems that affect your blood sugar levels, such as diabetes. This can increase the risk of diabetic ketoacidosis and other potentially harmful illnesses associated with drastic changes in blood glucose levels. When you break your fast, the drastic change in blood sugar can be dangerous. Being aware of what is happening inside of your body is key to approaching fasting healthily. Long-term fasting can be beneficial, but it should not be attempted if your body is not healthy enough for it.

Warrior Diet

One of the most extreme methods of intermittent fasting is the Warrior Diet. The Warrior Diet is based on a theory that humans are biologically built to consume and process food in line with their circadian clock. The diet consists of eating one calorically dense meal every evening and fasting for the rest of the day. This is based around the belief that "warriors" of antiquity spent their time fighting, hunting and generally taking care of business throughout the majority of the day, so they ate much less during that time. Therefore, they would end their days indulging in a larger meal. In this same way, individuals who practice the Warrior Diet fast for the majority of every day. Generally, this follows a 20:4 method, with a twenty-hour fasting window and a four-hour feasting window. During the 4 hours, individuals consume a high number of calories. This can lead some people to choose unhealthy foods, but it is recommended to eat a healthy, balanced meal, especially if you will be exercising during your fasting period. Fueling your body properly will help you get optimal results and stay as healthy as possible while practicing intermittent fasting. During the 20-hour fast period, you do not have to avoid food entirely. Small snacks made up of raw vegetables or fruits, boiled eggs, and dairy products are encouraged, and you can drink as many calorie-free beverages as your warrior's heart desires. This includes tea, coffee, diet sodas, and of course lots and lots of water.

The Warrior Diet was created by an ex-member of the Israeli Special Forces who found inspiration in his time as a soldier and carried his knowledge and experience into the field of fitness and nutrition. However, the creator of this diet admits that it is not based on science and the amount of research around it is nearly non-existent. This does not necessarily mean that it isn't effective, but it is a good point to remember when considering this method.

Many people who practice the Warrior Diet incorporate exercise into their routine during the fasting period. This can be an effective way to build muscle, but it carries potentially harmful side effects. Pushing the body to its limits when it is low on fuel (food) can cause fatigue and dehydration, as well as decreasing your overall ability to perform which may lead to injury. This can also lead to a condition called hypoglycemia which is essentially dangerously low blood sugar. Hypoglycemia can lead to problems of varying severities ranging from confusion, increased clumsiness, trouble forming words, and dizziness to seizures and possible death. If you have type 1 diabetes or are on medication designed to lower your blood sugar, you should never attempt this diet. Again, it is important to consult your doctor before trying to incorporate a fasting regime into your lifestyle. An extended fast such as this also increases the likelihood of binge eating and consuming foods that are not rich in the nutrients necessary to fuel the body. When you are consuming a full day's worth of calories in 4 hours, opting for a carb-heavy meal full of processed food may seem appealing. Ensuring that your body is receiving the proper vitamins and minerals to maintain its functions is crucial to a healthy practice of intermittent fasting. Incorporating a meal prep plan into your Warrior Diet can help to avoid this issue and increase your likelihood of success.

Practicing any method of intermittent fasting is not recommended for people who may suffer from eating disorders. Any restrictive diet is not suggested for people with a tendency to over-restrict calories. Also, most people do not use intermittent fasting as a lifelong commitment, so someday they will probably stop practicing it. After you become accustomed to fasting, eating on a normal schedule can cause unwanted weight gain. You may lose touch with your ability to sense when you are truly hungry or full, and you may become accustomed to eating higher calorie meals. If you are not careful, this may lead to overeating which can bring about feelings of shame or regret that can negatively affect mental health. In individuals who are at risk of disordered eating, the negative emotions connected to this can lead to bingeing and purging behaviors.

Depending on the state of your health, your lifestyle, your weight loss or muscle gain goals, and your reaction to fasting, there is likely a method of intermittent fasting that suits your needs. The 5:2 diet and time restricted eating methods like the 16:8 are ideal for beginners and have much fewer risks attached. If you want fast, drastic results, the Warrior Diet may be ideal for you. All of these methods will help you lose fat. Some will help you lose more fat, more quickly, and some will help you build and maintain muscle mass more effectively. You do not have to stick to one method forever. The beauty of fasting is that it can be done in whatever way suits your lifestyle the best and can be catered individually to your wants and desires.

5:2 Method

When it comes to the intermittent fasting methods that have several hours each day set aside to fast and the lingering hours set aside to eat, something gets lost in translation. Some people come to intermittent fasting with aims at big lifestyle changes, or with hopes of experiencing whole new timing and relationships to food. In that case, these individuals might prefer 5:2 method.

Like the crescendo method, 5:2 goes back to several days "on" and several days a week "off" when it comes to fasting. In specific, this method of IF (being more extreme than any others we've looked at so far) involves a severe restriction of caloric intake for two days a week and regular feeding the remaining five days. On the two restricted-intake days, the practitioner is only allowed 500 calories per day to maintain and actualize the goals of the fast.

If you're having trouble making 5:2 method work, try a different style of intermittent fasting altogether. It could be that this strange on-and-off method doesn't suit your lifestyle, and there are clearly enough other options that there's bound to be *something* that works just right for *you*.

Eat-Stop-Eat (24 Hour) Method

This method of fasting is incredibly similar to the crescendo method. The only discernable difference is that there's no anticipation of increasing (of "crescendo-ing") into a more intense fasting pattern with time. For the eat-stop-eat method, you decide which days you want to take off from eating, and then you run with it until you've lost that weight and then you keep running with the lifestyle for good because you won't be able to imagine life without it.

The eat-stop-eat method involves one to two days a week being 100% oriented towards fasting, with the other five to six days concerning "business as normal." The one or two days spent fasting are then full 24-hour days spent without eating anything at all. During these days, of course, water and coffee are still fine to drink (in fact, anything is still acceptable to drink during fasting periods as long as it's not too thick like a smoothie or protein shake), but no food items can be consumed whatsoever. Exercise is also frowned upon on those fasting days but see what your body can handle before you decide how that should all work out.

Some people might start thinking they're using the crescendo method but end up sticking with eat-stop-eat. The two are so similar. It's easy to see how this situation might occur. Furthermore, some others work *up* to the eat-stop-eat method from 14:10 or 16:8 methods. It could be that these individuals tried the daily fast window technique and wanted something more intense. Clearly, this method qualifies!

Alternate-Day Method

The alternate-day method is admittedly a little confusing, but the reason it could be so confusing could come, in part, from how much wiggle room it provides for the practitioner. This method is great for people who don't have a consistent schedule or any sense of one, and it is therefore incredibly forgiving for those who don't quite have everything together for themselves yet.

When it comes down to it, alternate-day intermittent fasting is really up to you. You should try to fast every other day, but it doesn't have to be that precise.

Alternate-day fasting is a solid place to start from, especially if you work a varying schedule or still have yet to get used to a consistent one. If you want to make things more intense from this starting point, the alternate-day method can easily become the eat-stop-eat method, the crescendo method, or the 5:2 method. Essentially, this method is a great place to begin.

The Warrior Method

The warrior method is incredibly similar to 20:4 method, but with one major philosophical difference, which makes this method all that much more interesting. The warrior method takes as its philosophical base the experience of the hunter/gatherer ancestors we evolved from. It's as if this method looks back at the origins of intermittent fasting and tries to make its example as historically accurate as possible.

In sum, warrior method involves fasting for 20 hours a day (although you can have one cup of raw, fresh fruit and vegetables dispersed throughout that 20 hours) and then eating one large meal during the 4-hour feeding window. Just like the warrior coming home from the hunt, the individual practicing warrior method will spend most of the day working (i.e. the fast lasts all day). Only to come home and focus on one large meal (i.e. the 4-hour eating window would always take place during the evening), from which the body can then extract all its necessary nutrients and proteins for energy, alertness, and fat burning.

Warrior method is the logical extension of 20:4 method when you want to take things up a notch of intensity (or of philosophical rigor). It can also be scaled back to 16:8 or 14:10 easily if you notice things just aren't working with this method for you. The biggest danger of warrior method is overeating during that one meal. To help protect against problematic overeating, make sure to have that one cup of fruit or veg as a snack throughout your 20-hour fast, and you can even try breaking up your big meal into smaller sections that are eaten across the 4-hour feeding window if things still aren't working out. If these adjustments don't curb the overeating, another method would definitely suit you better.

Chapter 17: Common Myths of Intermittent Fasting

When it comes to losing weight everyone seems to have their own two cents worth of advice to give. Even you have probably offered someone a tip or two about losing weight at one point or another. Today, information is available at the tips of your fingers. You can look up dozens of different weight loss programs on your phone, tablet, computer, in magazines, and books. Most of the time you can't go a day without turning on the television and seeing a commercial for a new "miraculous" supplement, waist shaper, or exercise DVD.

Fasting is Basically Starving Yourself

Possibly the greatest myth about fasting is that you are starving your body of food. Starving obviously isn't healthy and is attributed to serious eating disorders. But fasting is not an eating disorder nor is it starvation. In fact, intermittent fasting helps individuals develop stable and regular eating habits. Starvation is when you rob your body of food; you purposely do not give it any source of food, resulting in malnourishment and even death. Fasting is when the participant chooses select times to feed their body the proper nutrients it needs. Not only are you making better choices when you fast, but you are also giving your digestive system a rest. You cannot become seriously injured or die from fasting, because the point of intermittent fasting is that you do break the fast with a delicious meal.

Fasting Will Slow Down Your Metabolism

Your metabolism is the energy used to keep your cells active and alive, it sustains your life. While it is true that your metabolic rate effects your weight, intermittent fasting will not slow it down. Research has proven time and time again that the quantity of the food you consume matters, not your eating pattern. This means that how often you eat or when you eat does not correlate with your body composition. What really matters is how much food you eat in regards to your body composition and weight. Of course, when it comes to health, quality matters a great deal as well. Your metabolism is not a mystical fire that you should try to speed up. It is something that you should try to optimize. Fasting will not decrease your metabolism or put your body into starvation mode. Your metabolism will burn however many calories it can, and the only way it will burn more calories for energy is if you also exercise. As long as you eat in a caloric deficit and/ or exercise, you will lose weight.

You Will Gain Back the Weight You Lost After Eating

Another common myth is that fasting is a waste of your time because you will just gain back whatever weight you lose as soon as you stop fasting. The only way you will gain back whatever fat you lost is if you do not adapt fasting as a lifestyle and continuously eat after you stop fasting regularly.

Fasting Only Helps You Lose Water Weight

As with many diets, it is a common myth that when you lose weight you are actually losing water weight or muscle glycogen. While this does occur for some people, it is not necessarily true. You absolutely will lose weight in the form of body fat when you fast; it just don't be in the first two weeks of intermittent fasting. As long as you stick to your fasting schedule and plan, you will lose that stubborn belly fat.

Having Less Energy When Fasting

Some people believe that because you are eating less food when you adopt intermittent fasting, you experience a lack of energy. When you first begin fasting, you may experience a slight decrease in energy. But once your mind and body adapt to the change in lifestyle, you will actually have increased energy levels, even when skipping meals. The first week or so is the hardest, as it is with any other lifestyle change. When you are hungry, that is when you will expend the most energy. You can use hunger as motivation to stay strong in your goals and stay active and focused on other important tasks. If you keep yourself distracted throughout your fasting period, intermittent fasting is a much more pleasant experience.

Fat Makes You Fat

Many people choose to adapt much healthier diets when they take on intermittent fasting. One of the most common myths of losing weight through dieting is that eating fat will make you fat. But this is simply not true. Humans cannot live without fats; they are crucial for our survival. But there is a difference between good fats and bad fats. Good fats give us necessary fatty acids and vitamins, energize us, and keep our skin super soft. The combination of bad fats and carbohydrates is what makes people gain weight, not the consumption of fat. There are even studies that have shown a short term high fat, low carb diet will help you lose more weight than other typical dieting methods.

Your Brain Will Stop Functioning Without Carbs

Another myth about dieting and intermittent fasting is that if you do not consume carbohydrates every few hours, your brain will stop working. This belief comes from the theory that your brain can only use glucose to convert to energy. But your body can produce its own glucose through a process called gluconeogenesis. And your body has stored glycogen in the liver that can be used for energy. Lastly, long-term fasting or low carb diets will force your body to produce ketone bodies, which will also energize your brain. The fact of the matter is that our bodies are more than capable of surviving without a constant supply of carbohydrates. If this was not the case, humans would have been extinct long ago.

You Need Supplements To Make Up for Lack of Food

There are dozens of different supplements that "experts" claim your body needs during a fasting period. But you don't need green tea pills or raspberry ketones to lose weight and stay motivated during your fast. All your body needs is water.

Fasting and Training Are a Bad Combination

While some aerobic activities, such as running, may have a slight negative impact on performance, anaerobic performance, like lifting weights is not as effected by intermittent fasting. Although carbohydrates boost your energy while exercising, a key factor to a good workout is staying hydrated. The most common type of athlete that participates in intermittent fasting is a weight trainer or lifter. And luckily for athletes who are focused on changing their body composition, fasting allows your body to lose fat while still gaining muscle: as long as you feast with the right kinds of food.

Intermittent fasting will make you overeat, causing you to gain weight

Some people claim that you won't lose weight using intermittent fasting because you'll overcompensate during your eating periods and eat more than you would normally. This can be true, and some people do tend to eat slightly more after breaking a fast than they would have normally eaten had they not been fasting.

Chapter 18: Fasting to Lose Weight

If you maintain a healthy caloric intake during feeding hours, avoiding food during fasted hours will help you reach a caloric deficit. This means that you are consuming fewer calories than your body is using. To make up the difference, your body will use the energy in stored fat to fuel the processes it needs to sustain. Binge eating carb heavy, calorie dense, and unhealthy foods during fed hours can lessen this deficit, so for optimal weight loss, it is suggested that you also ensure that you are incorporating healthy meals into the equation. Decreasing the number of carbs you eat will avoid adding new fat stores. You'll be burning fat and also avoiding making more. Keeping insulin levels low will also help you burn more fat.

Food Choices

Fasting naturally lowers insulin levels and increases insulin sensitivity so your body will be absorbing sugars effectively. If you are consuming foods that cause insulin spikes, the body can start to store more fat rather than burning it. Wholesome, unprocessed foods are the most effective for avoiding this issue. When you go to the grocery store, the whole foods are generally located in aisles on the outside perimeter of the store. This is where you'll find fresh fruits, vegetables, and proteins. There are, of course, foods located on the inner aisles that can also benefit your diet, but the majority of a diet that will burn fat contains these whole foods. Knowing how macronutrients affect insulin levels will help you understand how to build your diet for optimal weight loss. Carbohydrates and dairy will have the largest impact on insulin because they are processed glucose. This means you'll want to avoid carbs as much as possible and lower your dairy intake. Proteins will have less of an impact on insulin levels. However, in the absence of sugars, the body will convert proteins into sugar using gluconeogenesis. Over consuming protein can cause insulin spikes as well, but less so than carbs. Fats have the least impact on insulin, so consuming more fats will fill you up without increasing insulin production. You can still incorporate dairy and carbohydrates into your diet without causing insulin spikes. Breaking your fast with a meal made of whole, unprocessed ingredients like vegetables will satiate your hunger so you can avoid overindulging in the more troublesome foods. Eat your vegetables and proteins first so that when you consume carbs and dairy, you will be doing so in smaller amounts.

The best way to be aware of what ingredients are going into your meals and ensure you are consistently consuming a healthy diet is to make the food yourself. This can be time-consuming. It can be difficult to work cooking into your schedule sometimes, especially if your eating window falls during the time of day where you are busy with work or other responsibilities. If this is an issue you come across, you may want to consider meal prepping. Meal prepping is the practice of taking a few hours on one or two of the less busy days of the week to prepare meals ahead of time. This does require a bit of an investment in both time and energy as it takes a large chunk out of the day, but the benefits it provides can help you to maintain a healthy diet, stick to your fasting schedule, and reach your weight loss goals.

The first step is to make a plan of what meals you want to consume in the coming days. It may help to make an inventory of the groceries you already have or to consider what foods you generally crave. It is also ideal to make meals that will refrigerate or freeze and reheat well as you won't be eating all the food right away. Once you've decided which meals you want to make, create a list of the ingredients you need. Choosing meals that contain common ingredients can cut down on the time and cost of meal prep. While shopping, remember the outer aisles of the grocery store are home to the more wholesome, single-ingredient foods.

There are two recommended fasting methods that may help you optimize your weight loss in a consistent, maintainable manner. The 5:2 diet is a great way to get started with intermittent fasting and is generally one of the less difficult methods to maintain over an extended period. The fact that an intake of calories is allowed even during the 2 fasting days may be helpful to your weight loss if you incorporate intense, fat burning exercise into your routine regularly. It's important to be aware of how you fuel your body, especially if it is being pushed to its limits. You can exercise during a fasting window that involves complete food avoidance and still be properly fueled, it just takes a little more planning ahead.

The other fasting method that may be ideal is a time restricted eating diet like the 16:8 method. This method involves fasting more consistently which increases the caloric deficit while also creating the benefit of a routine. It is, of course, not required that you follow a strict routine with any method, but the 16:8 diet allows the formulation of such. When trying to lose weight, building a routine can help you maintain the necessary consistency to achieve your ideal results. This does not just refer to the consistency in fasting, but also in eating healthy and exercising regularly. The more regularity you incorporate these aspects with, the more likely you will be to form healthy habits and achieve a maintainable healthy lifestyle that can positively benefit your weight loss and overall health. Other intermittent fasting methods will cause weight loss, and the results may be more rapidly visible, but these two types of eating schedules specifically can help you achieve healthy weight loss that is less likely to be undone if you stop practicing intermittent fasting.

Increasing the duration of your fasting window will also help you to burn more fat. After you become accustomed to fasting, carefully increase the duration of your fasting window. Fasting for 24 to 48 hours can increase the benefits of fasting exponentially. This should not be attempted in one drastic change. Gradually decrease the amount of time in your eating window by a couple of hours every week or two until you reach a point where you can fast for more than a full day. This will allow the levels of hunger hormones to decrease and enable you to fast longer without stressing your mind or your body too much. Extended fasting lowers insulin levels significantly and allows the body to burn more fat. A longer amount of time without consuming food will also increase the calorie deficit and allow for the use of more stored calories. Fewer meals eaten yields fewer calories added to the body. Some individuals think that decreasing the calorie consumption for a longer period will send the metabolism into preservation mode and decrease its effectiveness. This is based on the assumption that without adding calories to the body, the body will try to conserve the energy it has stored. Interestingly, the opposite happens. Noradrenaline production increases more with longer fasts. This can stimulate the metabolism by an increment of up to 14 percent. The body will use the stored glycogen it has and be able to metabolize calories more effectively when it is fed which will assist in weight loss. Noradrenaline also increases energy levels, alertness, and clarity in mental processes. This means that when you fast, you might expect to feel weak and depleted. Instead, your energy levels really aren't too terribly affected.

Exercise

If you choose to include HIIT workouts into your routine while fasting, make sure you are not doing too much. High-intensity interval training isn't named this way it is for no reason. High-intensity workouts should not be done every day. Most trainers who recommend HIIT encourage alternating high-intensity workouts with low impact, steady-state exercises (LISS) such as walking or yoga. On these days you can also focus on stretching or foam rolling sore muscles. You should also be sure to incorporate at least one, if not more, rest days where the body can focus on recovery. Some people choose to exercise during fasted hours to make the most of the fat burning state the body has already entered. If you want to do this, listen to your body. HIIT is high intensity. The idea is to push your body to its limits for a short period, then rest and repeat. Pushing yourself when you are low on fuel can be dangerous. It can lead to sloppy, incorrect body form that increases the potential for injury. You may also feel weak, lightheaded, or dehydrated. Drink plenty of water, and if you know, you will be doing HIIT during your fast you should ensure that the last meal you consume before beginning your fast is full of the proper fuel. Eat a large number of vegetables, a moderate amount of protein, and plenty of healthy fats. Also be sure to incorporate some carbohydrates, but not too much. These carbs will replenish the glycogen stores in the muscles to be used during your workout.

Step by step instructions on exercise during fasting

Individuals quick for an assortment of reasons including religious recognition, weight reduction and purifying purposes. In the event that you practice consistently, you might need to proceed with your exercise schedule; be that as it may, fasting implies you devour far less calories than you'd commonly eat in a day, which can make practice troublesome and even perilous. Understanding the rudiments of how to do adjusted exercise amid a quick, will enable you to remain dynamic while remaining safe.

Talk with your physician. You should see your specialist before starting any activity schedule, however considerably more when preparing to fast. Your specialist knows your medicinal history and can give rules particular to you. Tell your specialist about your want to fast and your activity design. They will have the capacity to let you know whether its harmful or good for you

In the event that you have any pain or uneasiness while working out or symptoms of fasting, end the fast and exercise and call your specialist instantly.

Your specialist's significant concern will probably be regardless of whether your heart is sufficiently sound for exercise while fasting.

Nutritionist's suggest not going lower than 1,200 calories every day when eating less when fasting, particularly on the off chance that you are vibrant.

Settle on a less hearty exercise. A low-force exercise might be more helpful in case you're fasting. This may help guarantee that your body doesn't utilize protein for fuel.

Amid a fast, your body depends on reserved vitality as glycogen (your body's stockpiling type of glucose). In the event that you haven't eaten in for a short time, you might run low on glycogen which will compel your body to utilize protein as fuel.

Pick exercise like strolling as opposed to running. Direct strolling is a low-power approach to strengthen your heart rate.

Do light yoga or Tai Chi. Moderate, deliberate movements not just adjust and invigorate the body, these old practices have been known to calm and clear the brain.

Garden or do light yard work. They require bowing, stretching and lifting, and other body developments. Both are fundamentally exercise camouflaged as a leisure activity or a fun errand.

On the off chance that anytime, notwithstanding during low-force physical movement, you feel woozy or mixed up, cease the activity instantly. You may need to drink water and eat a little dinner to enable you to rest.

Incorporate higher force exercise subsequent to eating. In case you're following an irregular fasting program or a fasting diet for weight reduction, you can in any case incorporate more lively power work out. Increase in the power or recurrence of your activity program is conceivable, yet it's best to do this on the days you've eaten.

Chapter 19: Fasting to Gain Muscle

Intermittent fasting has shown to be just effective as a normal calorie restrictive diet in many ways. However, people who choose the intermittent fasting route have been shown to preserve muscle mass when losing fat while groups following a calorie-restricted diet for the same period lost both fat and muscle mass. There are a few ways to optimize muscle gain while on an intermittent fasting diet. It is very important to remember to consult a doctor before implementing any fasting regimens into your daily routine, especially when the goal results involve drastic weight loss or muscle growth. The most important key is to ensure that you are eating enough calories during your fed hours to compensate for calories lost during workouts.

The primary differences between trying to lose weight while fasting and trying to gain muscle while fasting are the way you exercise and the food you eat. Intermittent fasting is a beneficial tool when trying to gain muscle because you can lose fat and build muscle at the same time. The fasting is taking care of the fat loss, so you do not have to worry as much about burning fat in your diet and workouts. This changes the way you approach training. Your focus isn't on toning up to look better, it's on pushing your limits and getting stronger.

Lifting Weights

To build muscle, you need to lift heavy. If you are new to lifting, you can get stronger by lifting at least 60 percent of the maximum amount you can lift for one repetition. If you are doing bicep curls and 45 pounds is the maximum amount that you can successfully curl only once, then you need to be using at least 18 pounds for each set of reps to be building muscle. 60 percent of a single rep max is generally an amount that you can lift between 15 and 20 times in one set. This is not a particularly heavyweight, but as a beginner, it will help you build muscle.

As your body adjusts to lifting weights, consistently it becomes more difficult to build muscle. Over time, you will need to increase the percentage to at least 80 percent of your max to still be getting stronger and growing muscle. This is going to be an amount that you can't lift as many times. Rather than being able to do 15 to 20 reps in one set, you are not likely to be able to surpass 8 or 9 reps before you can't do anymore. So, the amount of weight you lift will affect muscle growth.

Another factor to take into account is the speed at which you lift this weight. Many people encourage slow, deliberate reps when trying to get stronger. This may be helpful in maintaining proper form, but it is not as effective in building functional strength or optimal muscle growth. Maintain controlled movements, but lift the weight faster and lower it slowly. Lifting faster yields more optimal muscle growth results because it uses more muscle fibers. This increases the amount of damage to the cells in the muscles which in turn increases the number of new, healthy cells that are added to repair them. So, lift heavier weights and lift them faster, but always maintain proper form.

If you reach a point in your sets where you cannot complete the reps without cheating on your form, stop. Reduce the weight if you'd like to finish out the set, but do not continue if you can't do it properly. Not using proper form can cause stress and injury to the muscles. When you are lifting heavy, you are working your strongest muscle fibers. When these stop doing their part, weaker muscle fibers start to bear a weight they are not cut out for. Damaging the muscles is part of building them, but injuring them is not a factor we want to add to the equation.

Feeding the Muscles

Muscles grow when you feed them. When trying to add muscle while fasting, you will need to increase the number of calories consumed during the fed hours. On days involving exercise, make sure the body is fed a surplus of calories so it can have the necessary fuel to perform protein biosynthesis. During training, muscle fibers are damaged. The body is always clearing out old, damaged cells and adding newer, healthier ones, so these damaged muscle cells get replaced with new ones. The body also has a nifty skill called adaptability. It wants to become better suited to dealing with whatever stimulus caused the damage to muscle fibers, so when the muscles fibers are repaired the body adds extra cells. This causes the muscles to get bigger. This is why bodybuilding athletes consume so much protein. The goal is to ensure that the body synthesizes more protein than is broken down. If more protein is destroyed than is being made, you will begin to lose muscle mass.

When you are fasting to lose weight, the larger the calorie deficit you achieve, the better the results. When you are fasting and trying to build muscle, you do not want a large calorie deficit.

Instead, to gain muscle mass, you need to have a caloric surplus. This means that you'll need to increase the number of calories you eat during your feeding window, but that does not mean you should start stuffing your face with junk food to meet the necessary surplus.

Pay attention to the macronutrient levels in each meal to help you fuel your body in a manner that is helpful for your goals. Macronutrients include protein, fats, and carbohydrates. The ratio of macros that you incorporate into your meal plan can vary based on what diet you follow, but there are a few aspects that will be consistent across the board if you are trying to gain muscle. No matter what ratio of carbohydrates you incorporate into your diet, it is generally considered ideal to consume the majority of your carb allotment in your first meal after training. If you practice fasted training, ensure that your first meal after breaking your fast is the meal with the highest density of carbohydrates, contains plenty of protein and lower in fat. If you train during your feeding window, consume your carbs directly before working out for maximum muscle building benefit. Be sure to incorporate enough protein into your diet to fuel protein synthesis in the muscles to grow your lean mass. Eat multiple large, healthy and balanced meals throughout your feeding window to meet your macros and your calories.

What you eat is a huge part of any process where you are changing your body. It can sometimes be difficult to find the time to make enough food or eat frequently enough to maintain the calories you need to build muscle. Meal prepping large batches of food once or twice a week can ensure that you can spend more of your feeding hours eating to meet your macros and less time trying to prepare food. Find a day where you have an afternoon free and set aside that time to get your meals ready for the week. Think about what foods are dense in the macronutrients that you wish to consume so you can meet your goals easily and choose meals that will help you do so. Choose a few simple meals that you can make in bulk and eat repeatedly throughout the week to save time, money, and energy. Once you've chosen your meals, make a grocery list and ensure you have all the necessary ingredients.

It is important to know how glycogen affects the muscles and how to ensure that the body does not begin using muscle mass for fuel through gluconeogenesis when fasting. It is highly unlikely that the body will reach this phase during shorter periods of fasting, but in prolonged fasts, it may happen. Keep this in mind when choosing a method of fasting. Gluconeogenesis is the process of turning things other than carbohydrates, i.e., protein, into sugars when sugars are lacking. This process won't occur until the stores of glycogen in the liver and muscles are depleted which can take up to 24 hours but can take as little as 6 hours when exercise is incorporated. After an intense workout with heavyweights, glycogen stores in the muscles are depleted. Glycogen is made from glucose, i.e., sugar. To replenish glycogen stores, the body needs glucose. This is when a targeted diet comes in handy. This method incorporates consumption of carbs after a workout to re-up the glycogen stores in the muscles. This ensures that muscles continue to grow well. At the very least, ensure that on days you are working out heavily you eat a larger number of calories and incorporate enough carbs to fuel the glycogen levels in the muscles.

Once your body is accustomed to fasting, it becomes better at nutrient partitioning. This means the body starts to send nutrients to the muscles where they are needed rather than sending them into storage in fat cells. Pushing muscles to their limits during the fasted state ensures that glycogen stores are depleted fully, which allows sugars to be processed into glycogen to replenish the muscles rather than stored. This can be beneficial to muscle growth. Just remember, muscles have to be fed to grow. Even if you continue fasting after you finish your workout, be sure that the first meal you eat when you break your fast after your workout is your largest meal of the day. However, do not immediately consume this huge meal the moment you break your fast. This can overwhelm the body and spike insulin levels. Break your fast with a small portion of food, wait approximately half an hour, and then consume the rest of your meal.

Incorporating fasting when trying to gain muscle is beneficial because it increases levels of human growth hormone (HGH) and noradrenaline as well as increasing insulin sensitivity. HGH increases the development of muscle mass and protects it from deterioration. Working out in the morning when HGH is released into the body will improve muscle gains and help you recover better from your workout. Athletes since the 1980s have been known to use extraneous doses of the human growth hormone to increase their muscle gains and muscle retention. High levels of HGH like these can have negative effects on the body, but the levels that show in the body during fasting are high enough to be beneficial, yet low enough not to be risky. Human growth hormone is essential to the cell renewal cycle and stimulates the growth of new cells which can help in the protein biosynthesis of muscles when damaged cells are replaced.

The increase in insulin sensitivity allows the body to process glucose more efficiently. This means that, in essence, your body will start sending the nutrients from your food directly to the muscles rather than storing them as fat. This will help the muscles grow and help decrease excess fat storage.

Noradrenaline is also increased as a biological response to needing to find food. When you fast, the body thinks that food must be scarce, so it increases this hormone that stimulates mental clarity and increases alertness and metabolism of stored energy. In theory, if you were a starving caveman who needed to find food, you would have a boost in energy so you can go out searching for it. The increase in noradrenaline coincides well with increased insulin sensitivity because noradrenaline stimulates the release of glucose from the glycogen stores in the liver and muscles. This allows the glucose in consumed food to be metabolized into glycogen to replenish these stores which means less glucose is stored in fat cells.

Best Fasting Method

The list of fasting methods that allow you to gain muscle is a little shorter than the list that helps you lose weight. When you are just trying to lose weight, any method will be effective even though some are more effective than others. When you are trying to build and maintain muscle mass, any method that involves a fast longer than 16 hours is out of the question. When you fast, the decrease in glucose intake causes your body to start using stored glycogen. Anywhere after 6 to 24 hours, the glycogen stores in your liver and muscles are depleted. If you are trying to gain muscle mass, it can generally be assumed that you do strenuous exercise that will deplete glycogen stores much faster. When those glycogen stores are depleted, the body starts to get its glucose from gluconeogenesis which makes sugar out of protein. This protein usually comes from damaged cells as well as connective tissues and skin which generally means that incorporating fasting shouldn't raise concerns about losing muscle mass. However, when you are trying to gain muscle mass, this process can prevent you from having sufficient protein to build up the muscle fibers. After 12 to 16 hours of fasting, gluconeogenesis becomes responsible for

100 percent of the glucose maintenance in the body. If you are maintaining a protein-rich diet during the fed hours, this may not be much of a concern for a short while. However, consistently allowing the body to break down proteins for sugars over hours upon hours can prevent growth in muscle mass and raise the risk of eventually losing the muscle mass that you have already developed.

Alternate day fasting, the eat - stop - eat diet, and the Warrior Diet all incorporate 24 hour fasting periods are not beneficial to gaining muscle mass. The extended fasting periods increase the amount of time the body is utilizing gluconeogenesis, as well as creating a larger calorie deficit for the week. The 5:2 diet is also not beneficial because it does not involve a time where food is avoided entirely. This decreases the hormonal benefits of fasting, such as the increase in human growth hormone which stimulates muscle growth and the metabolism. HGH is suppressed during eating, so consuming even the reduced number of calories allowed on 5:2 fast days will not allow the desired increases in this hormone. Also, when we want to build muscles, we need an excess of calories to do so. Drastically decreasing the number of calories consumed for 2 days out of the week will create a caloric deficit. This could be combated by increasing consumption on the other 5 days of the week, but overall this method is not recommended.

The most highly recommended intermittent fasting schedule for individuals who desire to reap the benefits of fasting while also gaining muscle mass is time restricted eating, primarily the 16:8 methods. A fasting window of 12 to 16 hours will allow for the hormonal and fat burning benefits of fasting without being detrimental to muscle development. During the feasting hours, you should do just what the name says: FEAST. This does not mean to binge eat junk food, but you should eat often and eat largely. If you have trouble fitting enough food and calories into an 8-hour eating window, extend it by a couple of hours. Keep in mind that to build muscle you need a calorie surplus. If you'd like, you can fast following a 16:8 method for a few days out of the week and have an extended eating window on other days. The main goal is to ensure that for the week as a whole you have an average calorie intake that is greater than the number of calories lost. If you had a calorie deficit on some days, that's okay. Eat more on the other days to make up the difference.

Conclusion

Thank you for making it to the end of this book. I hope that you have learned some of the benefits and have a better understanding of how intermittent fasting, in some form or another.

The beauty of intermittent fasting is that it is more of a lifestyle as opposed to the common diet. Intermittent fasting is much less restrictive as it is focusing on when you eat more than what you eat. You can experiment with what fasting protocol best fits you and your lifestyle. Once you have adjusted to a schedule that works for you, there is nothing left but to enjoy feeling good and having the freedom to do and eat what you like. Intermittent fasting can and has helped a great variety of women to get onto the proper path for leading the healthiest life possible.

Remember that you are in control of your nutrition, health, and overall wellness. You do not have to follow intermittent fasting to achieve your goals, but this lifestyle is certainly a valuable tool to assist you with the health and physique you are striving for. Always remember that you are the one in control of what you eat and when you eat. If you choose to use intermittent fasting, that is a conscious choice that you are in complete control over. Never let any diet or exercise regimen gain control of you.

All the information that you need to follow an intermittent fasting plan is provided in this book. You can choose from any of the different variations of the diet until you find one that works well for you. Intermittent fasting is more of a change in your lifestyle rather than just a diet. If you want sustainable weight loss and want to lose fat along with it, then you should stick to this diet. You can see positive changes in your body within a month of following this diet.

Intermittent fasting is not only beneficial to your health, but it is also easy to follow.

Good luck.